Bakhtiyor Ergashev
Shakhzod Kamolov
Bekzod Ismadiyarov

CONGENITAL SMALL INTESTINAL OBSTRUCTION IN NEWBORNS

Bakhtiyor Ergashev
Shakhzod Kamolov
Bekzod Ismadiyarov

CONGENITAL SMALL INTESTINAL OBSTRUCTION IN NEWBORNS

(clinic, diagnosis and treatment

ScienciaScripts

Cover image: www.ingimage.com

This book is a translation from the original published under ISBN 978-620-8-01206-9.

Publisher:
Sciencia Scripts
is a trademark of
Dodo Books Indian Ocean Ltd. and OmniScriptum S.R.L publishing group

120 High Road, East Finchley, London, N2 9ED, United Kingdom
Str. Armeneasca 28/1, office 1, Chisinau MD-2012, Republic of Moldova, Europe
Printed at: see last page
ISBN: 978-620-8-19297-6

Contents

INTRODUCTION....4
CHAPTER I....5
CHAPTER II....11
CHAPTER III....23
CHAPTER IV....40
CONCLUSION....63
conclusions....66
PRACTICAL RECOMMENDATIONS....68
REFERENCE LIST....69

Бахтиёр Эргашев
Неонатальный хирург
Золотые руки
Кто спасает детские жизни?

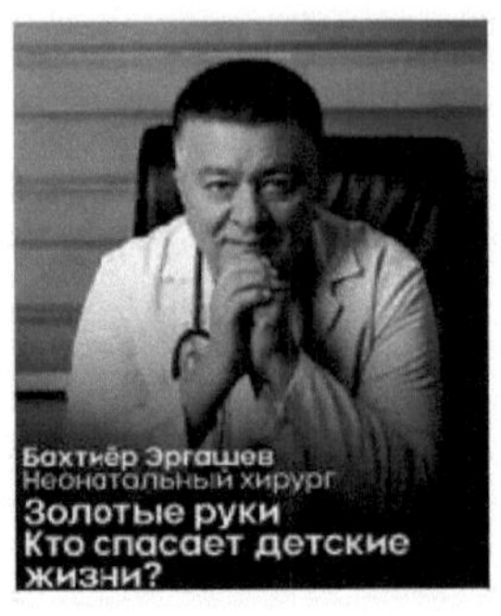

Bakhtiyor Ergashev - Doctor of Medical Sciences, Head of the Republican Training and Methodological Centre for Neonatal Surgery at the ROC, Professor of the Department of Hospital Children's Surgery, Tashkent Paediatric Medical Institute. He is the author of a successful operation on Siamese twins in the Republic of Uzbekistan and 10 methodological recommendations, 3 monographs, 2 manuals, 4 patents for invention and more than 150 scientific papers.
Scientific specialisation: Neonatal surgery, paediatric surgery, abdominal surgery, urology and coloproctology.

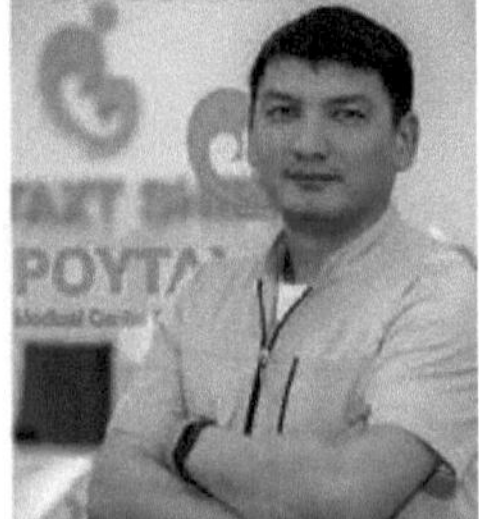

Shakhzod Kamolov is a candidate of medical sciences (PhD). Associate Professor of the Department of "Fundamental Sciences in the field of medicine" of Tashkent International Kime University. Physician of the highest category of the Republican Training and Methodological Centre of Neonatal Surgery. Author of 2 methodical recommendations and more than 20 scientific publications.
Scientific specialisation: Neonatal surgery, paediatric surgery, abdominal surgery, urology and coloproctology.

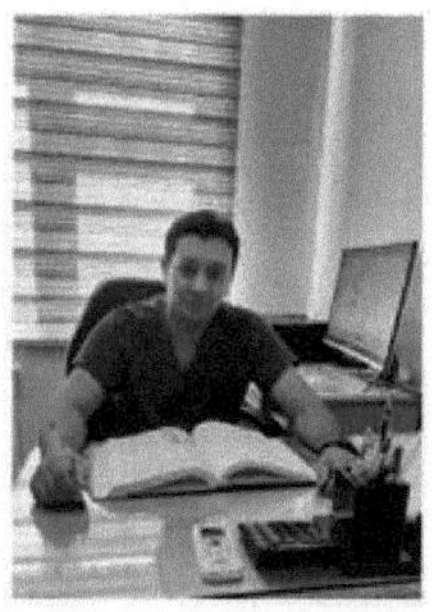

Bekzod Ismadiyarov is a candidate of medical sciences (PhD). Assistant of the Department of Hospital Paediatric Surgery of the Tashkent Paediatric Medical Institute. Physician of the first category of the Republican educational, therapeutic and methodical centre of neonatal surgery. Author of 2 methodological recommendations, 2 monographs, 1 textbook and more than 25 scientific publications.

Scientific specialisation: Neonatal surgery, paediatric surgery, abdominal surgery, urology and coloproctology.

INTRODUCTION

According to WHO data, of all congenital malformations, a quarter of all congenital malformations are GI diseases, in terms of frequency of occurrence they are on the third place, and complications of early postoperative period of these pathologies vary in a wide range from 9 to 77%, which reduces the functional efficiency of surgical interventions, and in 13% of patients forced to resort to repeated interventions for the purpose of reconstruction of the GI tract. Currently, to prevent severe complications of congenital malformations, the choice of treatment methods taking into account pathogenetic mechanisms and improvement of surgical tactics is one of the most important problems of medicine.

In the world, the percentage of children born with congenital malformations (CMD), despite modern achievements in science, is not decreasing and reaches 4.5%, with 25% being GI pathology, of which one third requires emergency surgical intervention during the first hours of life, and every fifth newborn dies from these pathologies.

The incidence of atresia of the small intestine (ATnC): jejunum (ATC) and ileum (IE) ranges from 20 to 50%, with an incidence of 1:1000 to 1:3000 neonates. It is often associated with other anomalies such as gastroschisis, omphalocele, and cardiac malformations. In 10.8% of cases, it is combined with pancreatic cystofibrosis and cystic fibrosis (Kumaran N., 2002), leading to the development of obturator KS, which in turn leads to a difficult postoperative period[14,121,130].

Therefore, a huge role is assigned to the diagnosis of GI malformations in the postnatal period. Timely diagnosis of these malformations after birth, assessment of morphological and clinical picture - all this determines the further tactics of patient management and will further improve the results of treatment of patients with GI obstruction. At present, during the newborn period, congenital small intestinal obstruction is the main cause requiring emergency surgery.

Thus, improving the quality of surgical treatment of ATNK and reducing postoperative complications and mortality in newborns by optimising prenatal and postnatal diagnosis and improving surgical treatment is one of the modern directions and is of great scientific and practical importance.

CHAPTER I

CURRENT ASPECTS OF CONGENITAL SMALL INTESTINAL (JEJUNOILEAL) OBSTRUCTION

During intrauterine development, the human intestine is laid in the form of an endodermal tube and differentiates into sections from the 4th week of the embryo's life. At the 5th week the primary mouth is formed, and at the 5th week the intestinal tube becomes multilayered, while the intestinal lumen is obturated and the stage of "dense cord" begins. The maximum rate of formation is found at the levels of the future duodenum and jejunum, where the vast majority of GI development anomalies are detected. Starting from the 6th week, the "vacuolisation stage" begins and by the 8th week the restoration of the intestinal lumen is completed. It is at this stage that atresia and stenosis may develop if the normal process is not followed [14,103].

In parallel, the normal intrauterine normal turnover of the "midgut" begins in the 5th week of intrauterine development and is divided into 3 periods The first period is characterised by rapid growth and lasts until the 10th week of fetal life. In the *second period,* the "midgut" returns to the overgrown abdominal cavity, which begins at 10 weeks and lasts until 12 weeks. The third period, up to birth, is characterised by a decrease in the level of the cecum to the right ileum and fixation of the intestinal mesentery [14,19].

The causes of GTCN can be divided into three groups: disorders at the stage of intestinal tube formation: atresia, stenosis, membranes; at the stage of midgut rotation ("rotation"); and congenital neoplasms leading to compression of the intestinal wall [2,16]. Intestinal atresia is usually formed in the first 3-4 weeks of intrauterine development when one of the above mechanisms is disrupted [46,82].

According to the literature, abnormal division of chromosome 22qll is a major factor in the development of intestinal atresia. The second mechanism is autosomal recessive inheritance. In addition, in 9-10% of cases, atresia is combined with cystic fibrosis; therefore, if a newborn with ATC and APC is found to have atresia, it is necessary to screen for the presence or absence of cystic fibrosis [14,30,62].

Some sources refer to a genetic theory for the occurrence of intestinal atresia: the relationship between congenital atresia and microRNA (ribonucleic acid) dysregulation [14,92,103].

Currently, there is also an ischaemic theory in the aetiology of this disease [7,8,36].

Diagnostic and tactical errors occur mainly in the antenatal period and ultimately affect the results of treatment of these patients. In the diagnosis of GNR during pregnancy in the initial period it is necessary to carry out a screening ultrasound examination (ultrasound), it is carried out in 3 stages: 3 stages: at 11-13 weeks - 1st trimester,at21-24 weeks - 2nd trimester, at30-34 weeks - 3rd trimester[40,62,63,126].

The presence of ATnC is indicated by the presence of dilated area of the jejunum at high forms of atresia. It should be remembered that several levels of fluid are detected, compared to DA, in which two are detected as a "double-bubble" symptom[14,51,95].

The presence of anovodia is also in favour of this pathology, but the degree is less pronounced than in DA. The method of measuring one free amniotic fluid pocket: an increase in the amount of amniotic fluid of more than 8 cm indicates hyperviscosity. Amniotic fluid accumulation may suggest proximal bowel obstruction as it is normally absorbed in distal parts[19,30,51]. Abnormal mesenteric blood flow in type IIIb ATNC can be diagnosed by colour Doppler examination of the mesenteric vessels late in pregnancy.

In the early diagnosis of GI tract anomalies in newborns, the most informative methods are radiology and intraluminal endoscopy, with the help of which it becomes possible to develop a surgical intervention plan taking into account the analysis of anatomical and functional features of the anomalously developed organ; to monitor the development of the pathological process in dynamics and to control the course of the postoperative period [30, 51].

A review abdominal radiograph confirms the diagnosis of ATnC in the postnatal period - the "double-bubble" symptom[14,55].

Irrigography is used only for the diagnosis of malrotation or in doubtful cases for differential diagnosis with other diseases with similarities to colonic atresia [126].

Abdominal ultrasound is necessary not only to confirm this pathology, but also to detect such a rare pathology - transposition of internal organs, as it will be necessary to make an abdominal wall incision in a different location [9,16].

Radiological signs of small intestinal perforation and intrauterine peritonitis are: "voluminous formation" of the abdominal cavity in the right half of the abdomen and on the opposite side dilated loops of the small intestine with multiple "levels" of fluid. A specific symptom of multiple atresia is the detection of meconium calcificates in the form of a "string of pearls" [51,56]. [51,56].

Currently, virtual endoscopy of the small intestine is informative for developing a plan and modelling surgical intervention [126].

Contrast computed tomography and shape modelling are appropriate when it is necessary to perform a CT scan of the neonatal body to confirm other combined malformations [14].

In some sources, it is stated that the degree of the affected area of dilated intestine and its extent depends on the level of the malformation: the lower the level of atresia, the more pronounced the destructive changes, which is confirmed by histological studies [83,84,145].

During the histological study, some authors (S.Suchithan et al. 2017) indicate the presence of intramural calcification and a pronounced reaction of giant cells of the foreign body in the sample of the atresiated area of the intestine and the adjacent area. It was concluded that there is a relationship between the histomorphological pattern and the size of the atresia site and the duration of ischaemia[48,145].

The classification of ATnC was originally proposed by L.W. Martin and J.T. Zerella (1976). Later, J.L. Grosfeld (1979) corrected it by adding a new type of obstruction - apple peel type anomaly and multiple ATnC[14,19,145].Today, the type of atresia ileal obstruction is determined according to the classification of J.L. Grosfeld classification

(Table 1.1.) [145].

Table 1.1.

Classification of atresia in ileal obstruction by J.L. Grosfeld.

Type of atresia	Characterisation
I	membranous (septal) atresia - has a membrane that completely occludes the intestinal lumen
II	Fibrous strand between proximal and distal segments: a pattern of dilated and hypertrophied proximal segment and hypoplastic distal segment with preserved length of the small intestine.
Sha	V-shaped rupture of the mesentery with non-critical shortening of the length of the intestine
P1B	atresia of the proximal small intestine with absence of the upper distal mesenteric artery, the distal small intestine is twisted like an "apple peel" or "Christmas tree". Newborns with this pathology are often premature with associated malrotation (50% of cases). Due to occlusion of the feeding artery is accompanied in most cases by extensive infarction of the intestinal tube as a result. Significant shortening of the intestine is observed in this case
IV	Multiple ATnCs in the form of a "sausage bundle" are represented by a combination of types 1-Sha and occur in 20-35% of patients with interstitial obstructions

There was also evidence of impaired muscle fibre thickness and contractility, changes in interstitial cells of Cajal in areas of the intestine above and below the site of atresia[32,33,145].

According to the theory of neuromuscular dysregulation disorders, Cajal cells may be important in the development of motor pathology in children of different ages, due to their association with intestinal stretch receptors [83,84,145].

The practical value of the above studies is that it helps to determine the extent of the lesion area that will need to be resected to prevent postoperative complications related to pathology from the histological structure of the intestinal wall[70,81].

German surgeon H. Braun in 1902 performed enterostomy for the first time on a newborn with ATNK. Thus, the development of various modifications of enterostomy began. For example, double intestinal enterostomy in children with ATCN proposed by Spriggs in 1910 led to death in 100% of cases [142]. Surgical intervention with the creation of a side-to-side interintestinal anastomosis in 1911 by P. Fockenso M. for ATNK was effective [81,142].

In patients with congenital intestinal malformations, necrosis and perforation J. Randolf et al. Randolf et al. proposed to perform enterostomy according to J. Mikulicz in 1940. Mikulicz in 1940. R. Hiatt and P. Wilson in 1948 for the first time performed enterostomy in newborns with meconial obstruction [137,142]. The creation of an

anastomosis with withdrawal of the diverting colon as a stoma was proposed by Bishop and C. Koorv 1957[37,79].
The technique of side-to-side interintestinal anastomosis with a proximal terminal jejunostomy was proposed by T. Santulli (1961), the use of which reduced the mortality of children from 80% to 62%. However, this method caused frequent problems with anastomosis patency due to kinking. The most advanced methods of surgery for these malformations are decompression "T"-shaped interintestinal anastomoses with a low risk of failure [79,142].
The technique of end-to-end anastomosis was proposed in 1967 by J. Louw. Louw, the dilated segment is resected and normal bowel is sutured to the distal obliquely crossed segment. With this technique, the survival rate reached 80% [130,142].With this technique, many surgeons prefer straight anastomoses, which do not create an obstacle to proper intestinal growth, do not lead to deformities and are technically easier to implement [10,26,92].According to some researchers, the end-to-end anastomosis technique is effective when the diameter of the intestinal loops is comparable [20,22,105].
In the correction of neonatal VTCN, a working intestinal union is necessary when there is a large difference in intestinal segment diameters, while traditional anastomoses have low efficacy due to failure and functional defects [62].
The technique of oblique anastomosis was proposed by I.V. Filipov et al. (2007). According to the studies of these authors, it is possible to create various interintestinal anastomoses in type IIIB and in the combination of types II and IV atresia. The following characteristics are in favour of this operation: minimal intestinal resection in the early postoperative period rapid restoration of intestinal function [56,57].
In type III-IV atresia, resection of the atresia and placement of a terminal end-to-end interintestinal anastomosis is the most suitable approach [78].
According to Williams et al. (2012), the most appropriate and length-preserving technique for ATK and AIC is the primary oblique or direct end-to-end intestinal anastomosis. This technique was tested on 30 newborns [139,143].
Adapted interintestinal anastomosis according to J. Louw is widely used. Louw with the frequency of sutures every 1 mm, which determines the absolute consistency of sutures and anastomosis [34].
According to V.A. Savvin et al. (2012), based on the experience of surgery of 42 neonates with ICH, it is considered that ATnC is the most physiologically applicable interintestinal anastomosis "end-to-end"[46,47].
Restoration of patency and bowel lumen is most expected when a primary interintestinal anastomosis is applied[105].
V.K. Patil et al. (2001), based on the results of treatment of 65 patients, recommend direct end-to-end interintestinal anastomosis with intestinal length preservation in all types of ATK and AIC. According to Ahmed A. Khalaf (2010), who applied this method in neonates with ATK and AIC, the results were disappointing: half of the patients had anastomosis failure, resulting in the death of the patients [105,144].

M. Machmouchi (2011) suggested resection of atresised bowel and insertion of a Foley catheter into the dilated proximal bowel to decompress and reduce its size [105,142] in multiple ATC and pagoda syndrome.

The Bishop-Koop T-shaped unloading anastomosis, which is the method of choice in ATNK combined with pagoda syndrome, relieves the load on the driving intestine for a long time in order to restore the functionality of the diverting intestine while minimising the loss of transit time of the intestinal contents[10,14,105].

There is a technique of T-anastomosis, which is applicable in ATNK - resection of the dilated driving part of the intestine and dilatation of the withdrawing part according to Wangensteen with the application of T-anastomosis, suturing according to Cherny and not intubating the withdrawing intestine, but in 55% of patients with prolonged syndrome of "non-functional driving loop" this method led to death [10,46,79].

Eduardo Branco-Blanchet suggested "T"-shaped interintestinal anastomosis according to SantullinpH in case of intestinal segments mismatch, intestinal perforation and perforation [18, 121]. In case of multiple ATnKWit J. suggested several anastomoses and the proximal part of the intestine is removed by a T-shaped anastomosis [79,98].

The first video-assisted anastomosis in a patient with ATNK (LAP-BAP technology) was performed by A. Yamatako et al. in 2004. Yamatako et al. in 2004: "through a semilunar incision along the upper edge of the umbilicus, a 5 mm trocar was placed and the proximal atresised end of the intestine was identified using endoscopic visualisation, after which it was extracted outside and an extracorporeal intestinal anastomosis was performed" [63]. [63].

This method was tested on 35 newborns by B. Li. Successful surgical correction without signs of anastomosis failure using laparoscopic anastomosis in newborns with ATNK on the second day of life was reported by Yu.A. Kozlov[105,142,145].

Postoperative complications and outcome.

In the new millennium, a high mortality rate of newborns with MVPD and decompensation of the cardiovascular, respiratory and urinary systems is also noted. Maximum early diagnosis of congenital gastrointestinal malformations is the key to reducing the number and severity of complications; preoperative preparation and competent transport are also of great importance [98]. Lethality in congenital low bowel obstruction is often due to septic complications as a result of late diagnosis, with newborns hospitalised and operated on for peritonitis, immaturity and prematurity[149].

Inter-intestinal anastomosis failure occurs in 5-10% of patients, and SCC and adhesion obstruction are frequently reported in survivors [94].

The survival rate of neonates with ATNK without complications tends to 100%. Among severe patients with IIIb and IV atresia, mortality is about half due to SCC and severe malabsorption [59,60].

Postoperative mortality rates for congenital small bowel atresia are distributed differently in different regions, for example: in India in2017 - 15.1%, in Russia in 2019. - 21.7-25%.,in Africa 2020. - 50.1%, in Ukraine in2021 - 42%.

The analysis of literature shows that single publications of domestic and authors from neighbouring republics confirms the poor study of this problem as a whole in the Central Asian region and indicates the need to improve the diagnosis and treatment of EIA.

Summary of the chapter

Thus, the analysis of literature data on modern aspects of embryogenesis, epidemiology and diagnosis of UTI shows that the discussion of criteria for antenatal diagnosis of fetal EIA is extremely important, early ante- and postnatal diagnosis, adequate assessment of the severity of children with small intestinal obstruction at different stages of treatment, taking into account the combined anomalies, concomitant somatic pathologies and complications has not only theoretical but also practical importance and requires the development of new methodological positions.

The high incidence of postoperative complications requires improvement of the methods of surgical correction of this malformation. The main causes of lethal outcomes in neonates with VTCN are associated with late diagnosis of the pathology and immaturity of the patient.

An integrated approach to pre- and postnatal diagnosis and treatment of neonatal ileal atresia would allow us to develop a comprehensive understanding of the pathogenesis in the pre-, intra- and postoperative periods, possible surgical complications and improve the results of correction of this malformation.

CHAPTER II

CLINICAL CHARACTERISATION OF THE MATERIAL AND RESEARCH METHODS.

2.1.General characterisation of the clinical observations

The work was carried out on the basis of the Republican Training and Methodological Centre for Neonatal Surgery under the ROC, at the Department of Hospital Children's Surgery of the TashPMI.

The present work is based on the results of diagnosis and treatment of 113 newborns with ATC and ACE at the RCHS from 2014 to 2021. During this period, 273 newborns with congenital obstruction of the small and large intestine were operated on at the centre. Among the malformations of the small intestinal tube, atresia predominated in 113 (41.4%), less frequently - stenosis in 12 (4.4%), disorders of intestinal rotation and fixation in 23(8.4%), meconium ileus in26(9.5%), other malformations in the large intestine (stenosis, NEC, etc.) in 99(36.3%) cases, respectively. Thus, atresia was observed in the majority of children admitted to our centre with a diagnosis of congenital atresia.

obstruction of the lower intestine. This was the reason for choosing the topic of our thesis.

During this period, 2799 children with various organ and systemic CHD were admitted, among them 113 (4%) with EIA (Fig. 2.1).

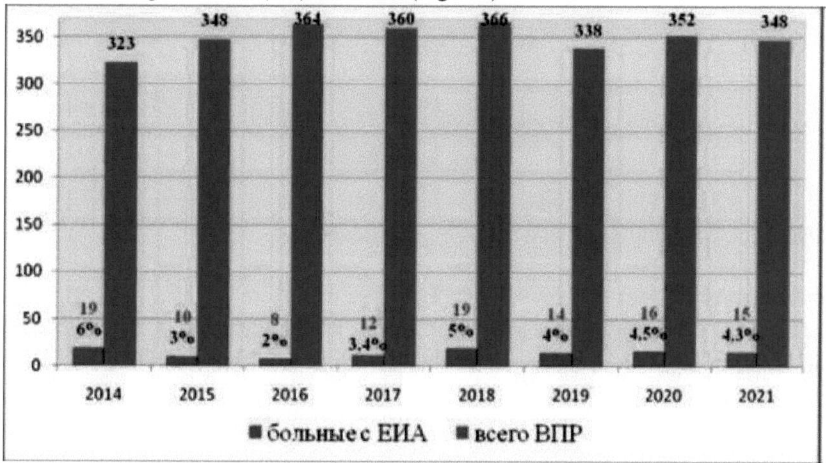

Fig.2.1: Dynamics of children with different IDTs and EIAs

Out of 113 neonates with congenital EIA, boys were - 57 (51%) and girls were - 56(49%) (Fig.2.2).

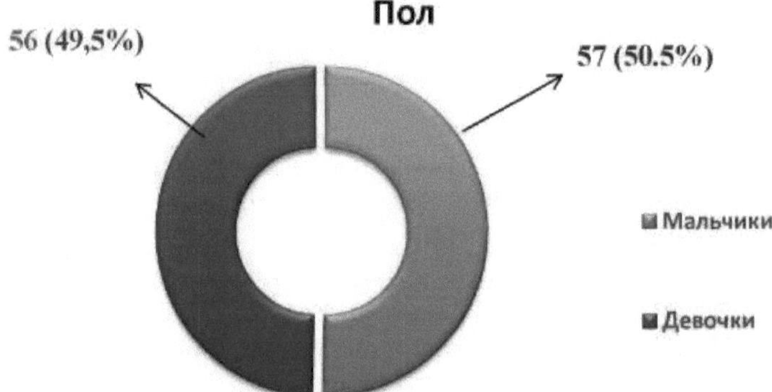

Figure 2.2. Distribution of patients by sex

Preterm babies (by gestational age) were 70 (62%) and premature babies were 43 (38%) (Figure 2.3).Of these, Grade I prematurity was 27 (23.9%), Grade II and III -15 (13.2%), with critical birthweight
was 1 (0.9%) (Figure 2.3).

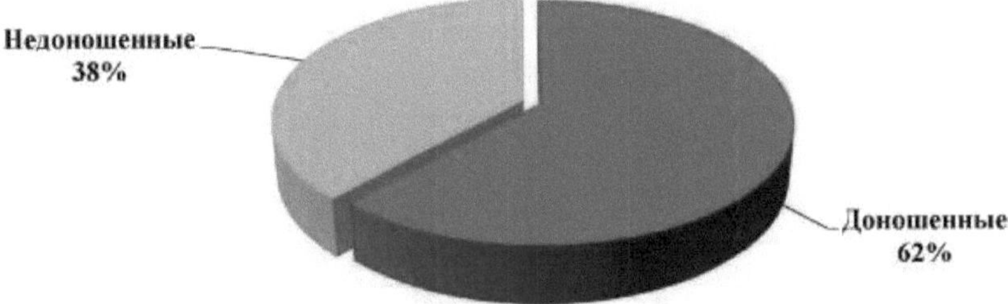

Figure 2.3. Distribution of newborns by gestational age

As can be seen from the above data, EIA was partly more frequent among male children (57%), and by gestational age, preterm babies prevailed (62%). Our study shows that the number of children born at 38-40 weeks is the majority (Fig. 2.4).

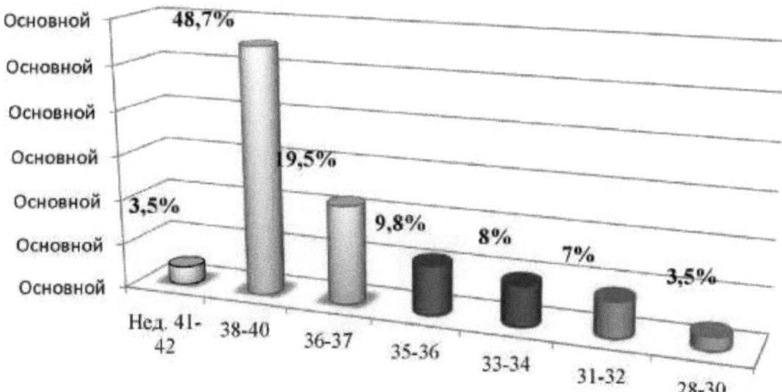

Fig. 2.4.Distribution of children according to gestational age

Newborns with congenital EIA were included in the studied group of GIACD. This is due to the fact that this GI malformation is more common than other GI malformations (NEC, DN, colonic obstruction, stenoses, lumen compression by abnormally located vessels, fetal tracts, abdominal tumours) and requires urgent surgical treatment in the first hours after birth (Fig. 2.5).

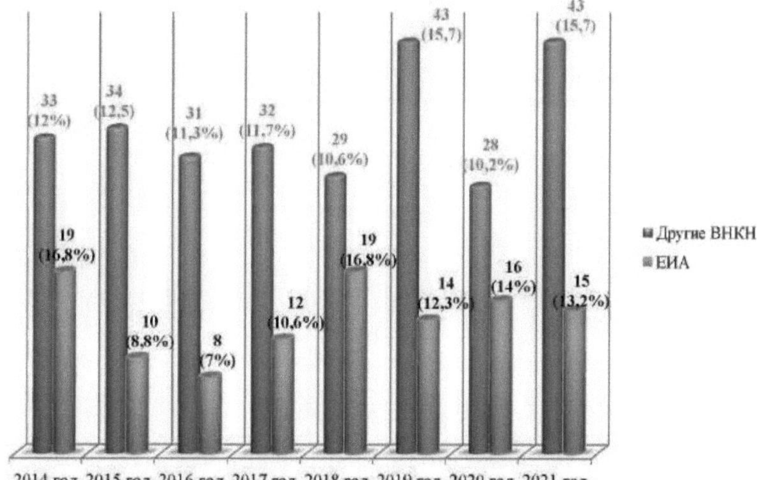

Fig.2.5: Dynamics of enrolment and ratio of newborns with congenital ICH and EIA

The examination of newborns with GI tract abnormalities before admission to the surgical hospital included: physical diagnosis; gastric probing; chest and abdominal radiography; and monitoring of blood, urine, and acid-base parameters.

All 113 (100%) newborns were examined under this programme.

Gastric probing is recommended in all patients with suspected congenital abnormalities of the intestinal tube. If more than 25-30 ml of greenish or yellow coloured liquid is obtained through the probe, the localisation of the defect in the duodenum or early jejunum is suspected.

Most patients came to the centre with the following complaints: absence of stools, abdominal bloating, vomiting with bile, ICH symptoms.

The primary diagnosis of VTCN in 68(60%) neonates with typical symptoms was made at the centre (Figure 2.6.).

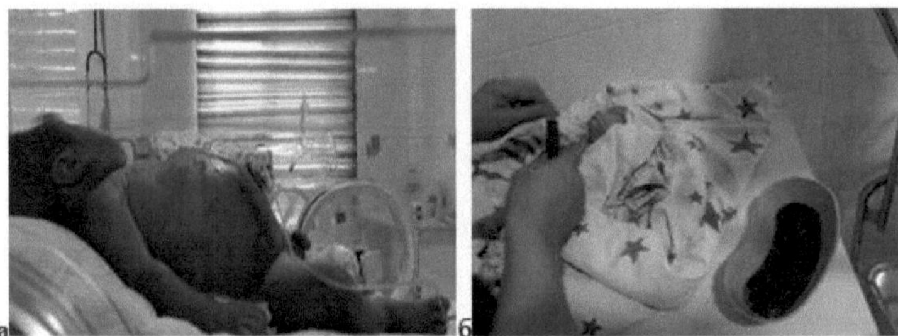

Fig.2.6.Appearance of the newborn: a) patient R.S. I.B.#208. bloated abdomen. b) patient I.S. #220. vomiting with admixture of bile.

NSCLC is characterised by the absence of meconium, instead of which scanty mucous masses are secreted from the rectum. In our observations, the main symptom of this malformation was a "mucus plug" in 111 (98%) newborns (Fig. 2.7.).

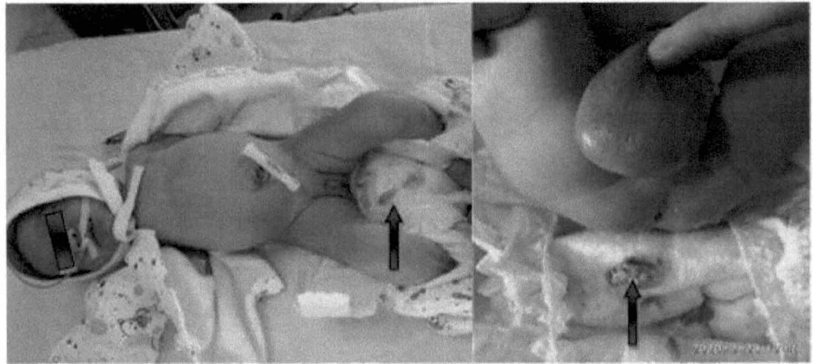

Fig.2.7. Patient D.S. I.B. #397 and patient E.M. I.B. #17. After stimulation of the rectum with hypertonic solution (microclysms), "mucous plug" was excreted in newborns

45(40%) newborns were admitted to the admission department of the RCHS with a previously established diagnosis or to clarify the primary diagnosis (Figure 2.8.).

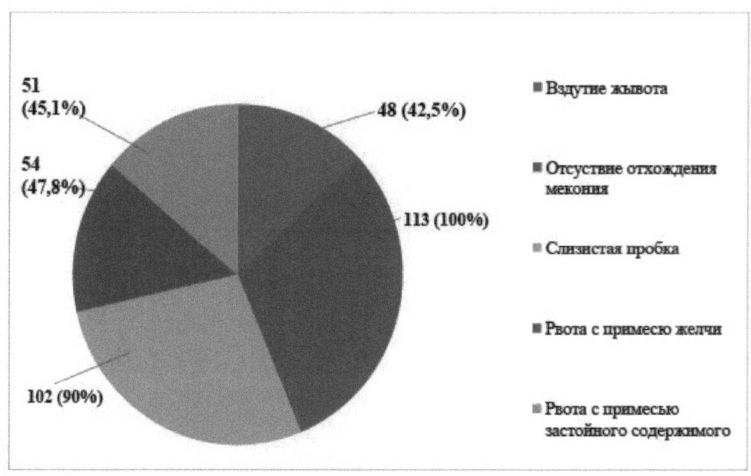

Abdominal bloating Absence of meconium discharge
Mucous plug
Vomiting with bile.
Vomiting with stagnant contents

Fig.2.8 Frequency of typical symptoms of VTCN in newborns (n=113)
We used the **classification of EIA** according to J.L.Grosfeld (1979). Today **The type of jejuno-iliac atresia is determined according to this classification, according to which there are 5 main types of atresia: I, II, IIIa, IIIb,** 1U (Fig. 2.9).

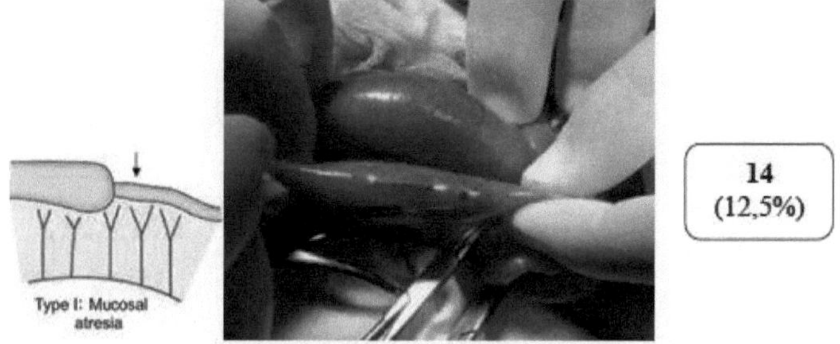

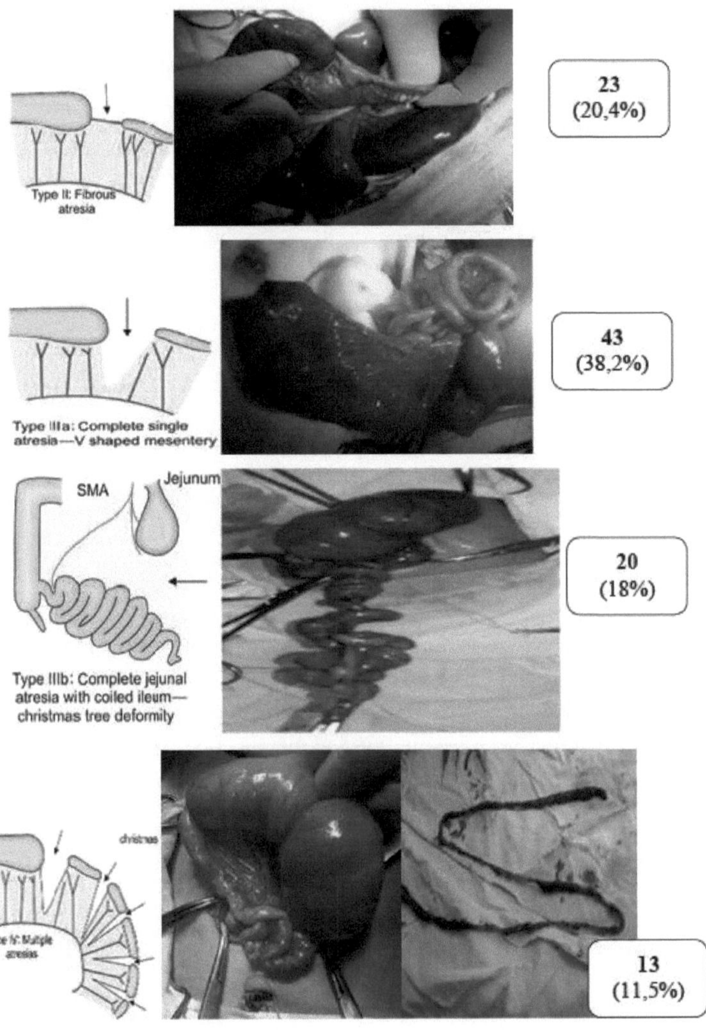

Figure 2.9. Schematic and clinical types of ATC according to J.L. Grosfeld classification. Grosfeld (brief explanation is written in English) I type - patient M.D. I/B No. 807, II type - patient M.M. I/B No. 1015, IIIa type - patient A.M., I/B No. 619, IIIb type - patient R.W. I/B No. 580, IVrnn - patient A.M. I/B No. 294.

Membranous or septal form of small intestine-type I was found in 14 (12.5%) neonates. Type IIIA of the small intestine was detected in 23 (20%) cases; type IIIa in 43 (38%) cases, type III6 in 20 (18%) and type IVIA in 13 (11.5%) neonates (Fig. 2.10.).

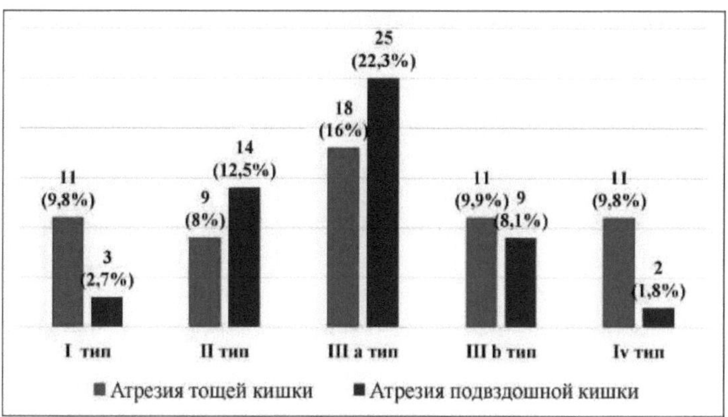

Fig.2.10. Comparative characterisation of patients by type

In our study, extragenital pathology was predominant in 41 (36%) cases and aggravated obstetric and gynaecological history in 26 (23%) of pregnant women. Factors aggravating the course of pregnancy - in 64 (56.6%) cases, social factors - in 69 (61%). Complications in labour were observed in 25 (22%) cases, caesarean section in 24 (21.2%) cases.

All pregnant women in the risk group for congenital fetal pathology were examined at the perinatal centre with mandatory consultation with a geneticist and obstetrician-gynaecologist, repeated blood tests for alpha-fetoprotein (AFP), fetal ultrasound with Doppler (Fig. 2.11).

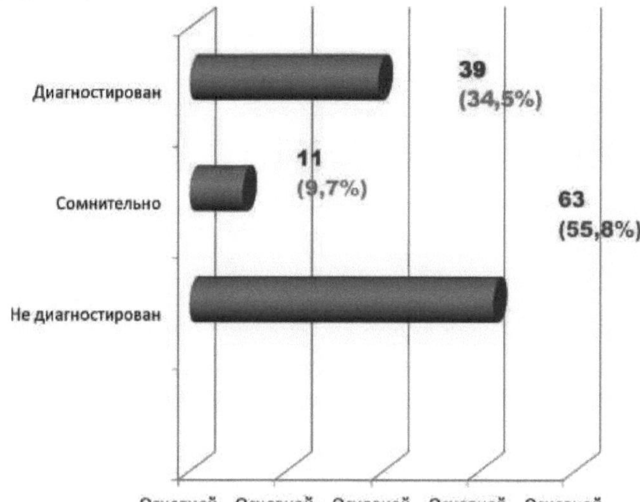

Fig.2.11. Detection of ICH at ultrasound in antenatal period (n=113)

Individual exchange charts of pregnant women and medical records of newborns were analysed. In addition, the data of genetic testing and the materials of the emergency mobile counselling department were analysed.

The age of women who had neonates with congenital ileal obstruction averaged 23.4±5.6 years, of which women under 17 years of age in 3(2.7%), 17-25 years in 54(47.8%), over 34 years in 56(49.5%) cases respectively.

When collecting anamnestic data from pregnant women with fetal VTCN, the following diseases were detected: anaemia in 79 (70%) women, thyroid diseases in 11 (9.7%), neurocirculatory dystonia (NCD) in 26 (23%), refractive disorders (myopic refraction) in 4 (3.5%), chronic inflammatory diseases of the urinary system in 28 (24.7%), and viral diseases in 89 (78.7%) women.

Aggravated obstetric history was observed in 59 (52.2%) cases: previous abortions for medical reasons in 25 (22.1%), miscarriages in 10 (8.8%) cases, neonatal death in 14 (12.4%) cases.

The course of pregnancy was complicated by: threat of abortion in 79 (70%), genitourinary tract infection in 39 (34.5%), fetal hypotrophy in 3 (2.6%), intrauterine fetal hypoxia in 56(49.5%) cases respectively.

The main echographic sign of ATNC is considered to be the presence of dilatation of the intestinal loops, which is visualised by multiple "bubbles" in the fetal abdomen (Fig. 2.12).

Increased amniotic fluid volume is a recognised risk factor for preterm birth (in ATK - 20% of cases, in APC - 66% of observations).Of the 113 pregnant women, multigestation was determined indirectly by ultrasound criteria, usually using the amniotic fluid index (AFI (or AFI) normally ranges from 5 to 24 cm). Eighty-nine (78.7%) pregnant women were found to have multiple pregnancy (Figure 2.12).

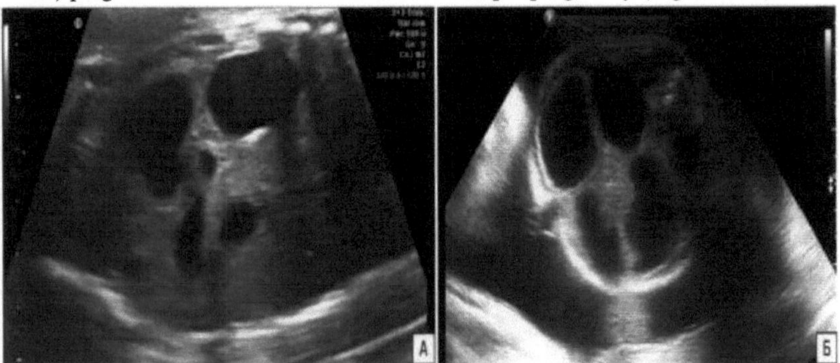

Figure 2.12. Cross-section of the fetal abdomen at ATnC: pregnant E.B. I.B. #404. a). 27 weeks of gestation. b). 29 weeks of gestation.

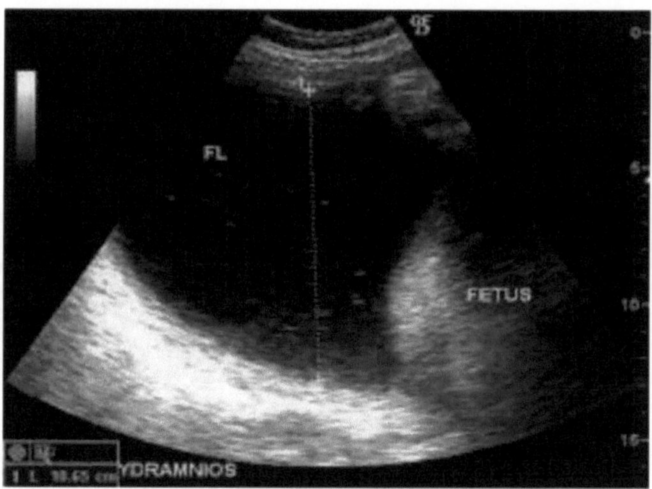

Figure 2.13.Polyhydramnion at 32 weeks of gestation

All pregnant women at our centre were examined by gynaecologists for general physical and clinical examination, including somatic and obstetric-gynaecological anamnesis, gynaecological examination, determination of blood group and Rh factor, clinical blood and urine tests, oestriol level, and smear for purity. After these examinations, which were concluded after a consilium of our doctors for termination of pregnancy for medical reasons on the fetal side at 20-22 weeks gestation, 8 (16%) pregnant women were found to have uncorrectable malformations (3 (37.5%) with anencephaly, 4 (50%) with spinal cleft and 1 (12.5%) with hydrocephaly).

2.2 Characteristics of the methods of investigation of newborns with VTNC.

To diagnose VTCN, we performed the following methods of investigation.

1. ***Laboratory examinations*** on admission to the clinic:

- Complete blood count, clotting time; blood type;

-biochemical blood analysis: total protein, urea, bilirubin, glucose level, C-reactive protein; coagulogram; total urine analysis;

Anaemia was detected in 16 (14.1%) newborns. The haemoglobin level averaged 114 g/l with minimum values up to 106 g/l in newborns with VTCN. In blood biochemical analysis, hypoproteinaemia was detected in 13 (11.5%) children; SRB elevation - in 26 (23%).

2. ***Ultrasound examinations*** included sonography of internal organs, neurosonography (NSG), echocardiography (Echocardiography) and fetal ultrasound.

Ultrasound of internal organs and *NSG* were performed on 92 (81.4%) newborns according to the standard technique on a Canon Xario 100 device using 3.5-7.5 MHz convex and linear transducers.

EchoCG was performed in 78 (69%) patients using ultrasound device "Aplio 500" of "Toshiba" company with cardiological paediatric sector transducer 2.5-6.5 MHz in the mode of colour, pulse, continuous-wave Dopplerography in real time.

Fetal ultrasound examination was performed on all pregnant women during the gestational period. 28 (24.8%) pregnant women underwent this examination at the RTC using Aloka SSD-1400 with convex, microconvex and linear transducers of 3.5-5-7.5 MHz. The most indicative sign of high level small bowel obstruction is multivaginal obstruction (Fig. 2.11. a). Fetal small bowel obstruction was diagnosed by the presence of multiple dilated bowel loops (more than 15 mm) (Fig. 2.14).

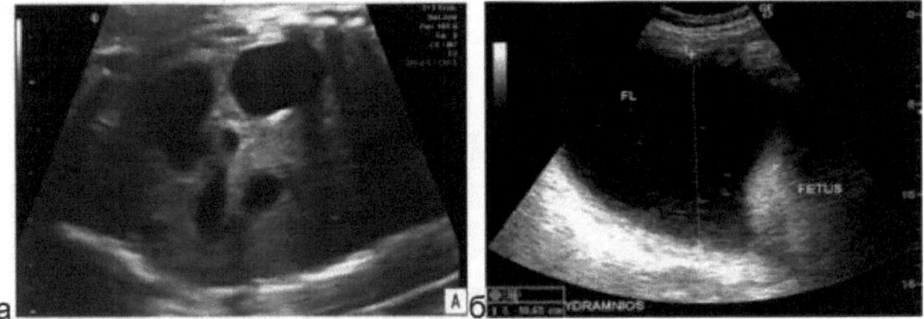

Fig.2.14 Fetal ultrasound: a) echo picture of dilated small intestinal loop up to 20 mm; b) polyhydroamnion in the foetus

Hyperechogenic bowel is a term that refers to an increase in the echogenicity (brightness) of the bowel on an ultrasound image. The finding of hyperechogenic bowel is not a malformation of the bowel, but a reflection of the nature of its ultrasound image. It should be remembered that the echogenicity of normal bowel is higher than the echogenicity of neighbouring organs (liver, kidneys, lungs), but such bowel is not considered hyperechogenic. Only a bowel whose echogenicity is comparable to that of fetal bones is considered hyperechogenic (Figure 2.15).

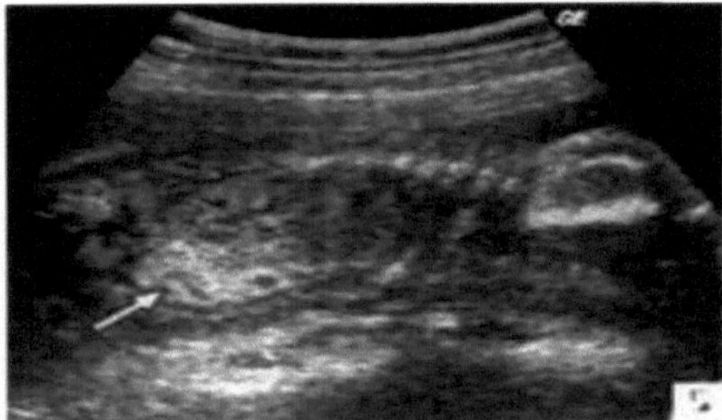

Figure 2.15: Increased echogenicity of the foetal intestine in the second trimester ultrasound of pregnancy

Radiological studies. Direct radiography of the abdominal cavity in the upright position made it possible to determine a significant increase in the size of small intestinal loops, their different filling with gases and the presence of fluid levels in them against the background of a normal picture of the large intestine. An increase in the number of visualised bowel loops indicates distal obstruction (Fig. 2.16.).

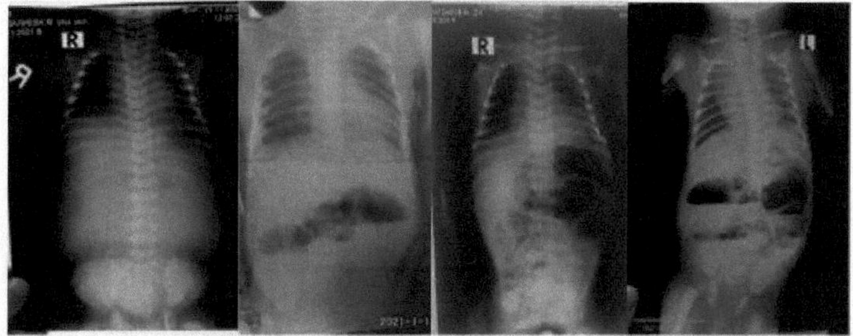

Fig. 2.16. Types of abdominal overview radiographs for VTCN in neonates on admission to RCHS.

This radiological picture is absolutely reliable and does not require additional methods of investigation, including the use of contrast. The more distal the atresia, the more levels in the intestine. In case of doubtful clinic and radiographs or when determining concomitant malformations, we use additional methods of investigation.

The traditional device examination is *radiography with contrast.* In doubtful cases, we performed GI passage in 31(27.4%) newborns. Triombrast 76% was used for this purpose. By intravenous administration, it enters the small intestine after 15 min. After another 1 h, the progression of contrast through the small intestinal lumen allows us to assess its configuration and identify the blind end (Fig. 2.17).

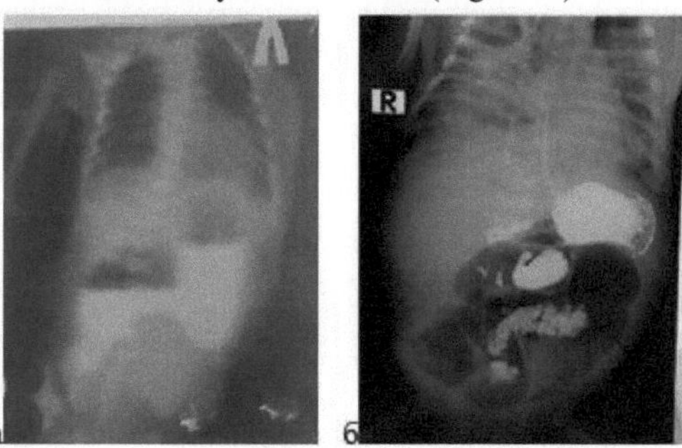

Fig.2.17. GI tract passage in VTCN in newborns on admission to RCHS a) atresia in the initial part of the small intestine; b) in the lower part of the small intestine

Irrigoscopy was performed in 64 (56.6%) patients. We do not recommend the use of barium suspension in contrast irrigoscopy. At irrigography with water-soluble contrast, so-called barium stones are not formed. It is easier to inject, unlike barium, it does not clog the probe, soaks the mucous mass, allows to remove the mucous mass from the rectum and gives information about the rectum. Low congenital intestinal obstruction is diagnosed with the examination. A microcolon is detected, on the mucosa of which characteristic folds are not contrasted, narrowing of the intestine, pronounced gaustration, positive symptom "small intestine" (Fig.2.18).

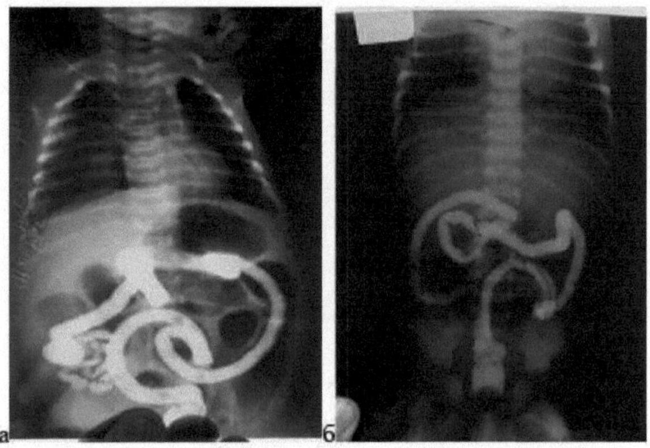

Fig.2.18. Types of irrigoscopy for neonatal UTIs
on admission to RCHS

The images can assess the shape of the intestine, its location in the abdominal cavity and length, its ability to stretch, elasticity, and the state of natural flaps and constrictions. An absolute contraindication to irrigoscopy was the suspicion of intrauterine peritonitis in a newborn.

Statistical processing of the research material

Statistical processing of the study results was carried out by methods of variation statistics using the program "Statistica 7.0 for Windows" (StatSoft inc., USA) calculating the mean and arithmetic mean error by the method of moments (M±m),mean square deviation (c) at normal distribution of signs and non-parametric methods to analyse the relationship of qualitative signs - x .^{2}

To determine the statistical significance of the obtained measurements we used Student's difference criteria (t) and degree of confidence (P) for data with normal distribution, differences were accepted as reliable at 95% confidence interval ($P<0.05$).

CHAPTER III

ANALYSING THE RESULTS OF DIAGNOSIS AND TREATMENT OF SMALL INTESTINAL OBSTRUCTION AND MEASURES TO IMPROVE THEM

2.1. Clinical characteristics of children with EIA

Clinical signs of jejunoileal atresia were noted as early as 1 day after birth: absence of meconium (100%), presence of "mucus plug" (100%) (Fig. 3.6 a.).

For the first 24 hours of the newborn's life, his condition worsened - restlessness and crying increased, intoxication intensified - lethargy and adynamia increased, and the skin became greyish-earthy. Doctors recorded uniform abdominal bloating with loops of small intestine identified on the anterior abdominal wall (Fig. 3.1.b.).

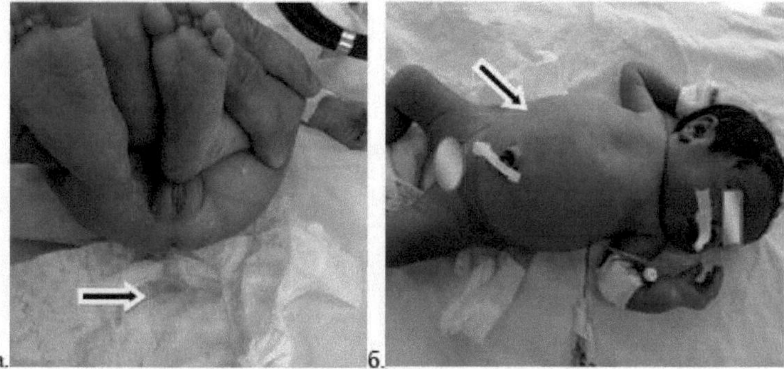

Fig.3.1 Patient Zh. 16.02.2019, born 16.02.2019 #178 with VTCN. a) rectal stimulation revealed a "mucous plug" b) examination revealed abdominal bloating

Congestive vomiting appeared, becoming meconial over time (Figure 3.2).

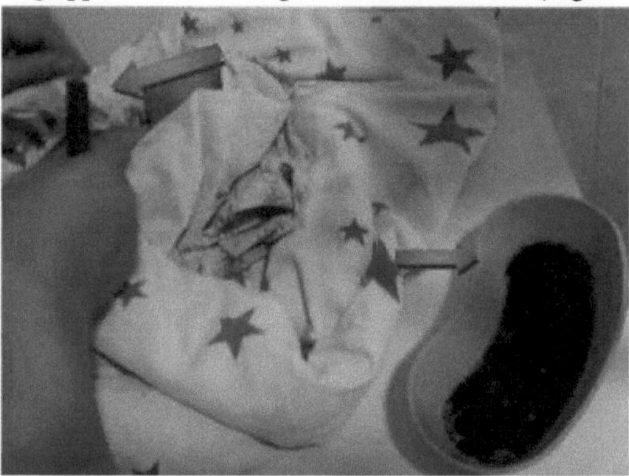

Fig.3.2 Patient Zh. 16.02.2019 year of birth #178 with VTCN. During gastric decompression, pathological secretion is released

On examination, the abdomen was soft, sensitive, moderately painful (enlarged bowel loops). At the beginning of the disease, rare muffled peristaltic noises were heard on auscultation, which were absent due to progressive intestinal paresis in the later period.

Abrupt deterioration with the development of signs of shock indicated the development of a complication: intestinal perforation and/or the development of faecal peritonitis: swelling of the abdominal wall, redness and/or cyanosis of the skin around the umbilicus, abdominal wall tension and sharp tenderness on palpation, no intestinal peristalsis was heard on auscultation (Fig.3.3).

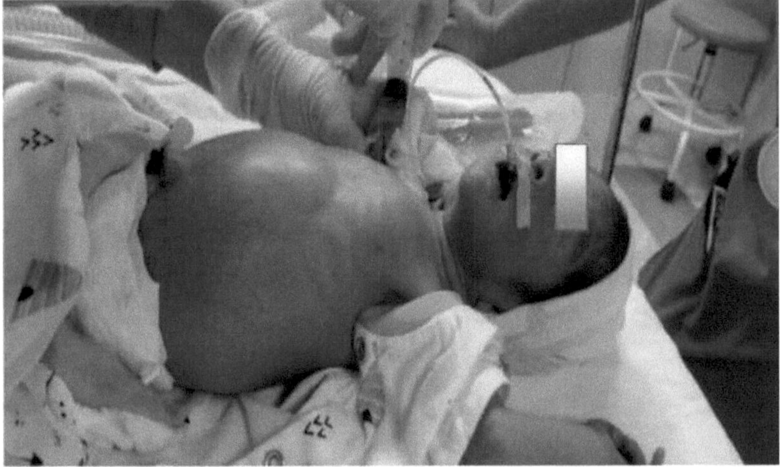

Fig.3.3 Patient U. (f.m.) I/B. No. 312 with perforative peritonitis (skin marbling and hyperaemia around the navel)

Radiological examination (review radiographs of the abdominal cavity) as one of the main methods of diagnostics of VTCN was performed in all 100% of patients. Radiological examination was started with review radiographs in the upright position. In low intestinal obstruction, the review radiographs revealed increased gas filling of intestinal loops, dilated loops, and sometimes the presence of levels (Fig. 3.4.). In 105 (92.9%) cases, we limited ourselves to review radiography, which showed VTCN. Gas filling of the underlying abdominal cavity was absent. The presence of free gas in the abdominal cavity and fluid level indicated intestinal perforation.

It is assumed that the more air in the intestine, the lower the localisation of atresia (Figure 3.4).

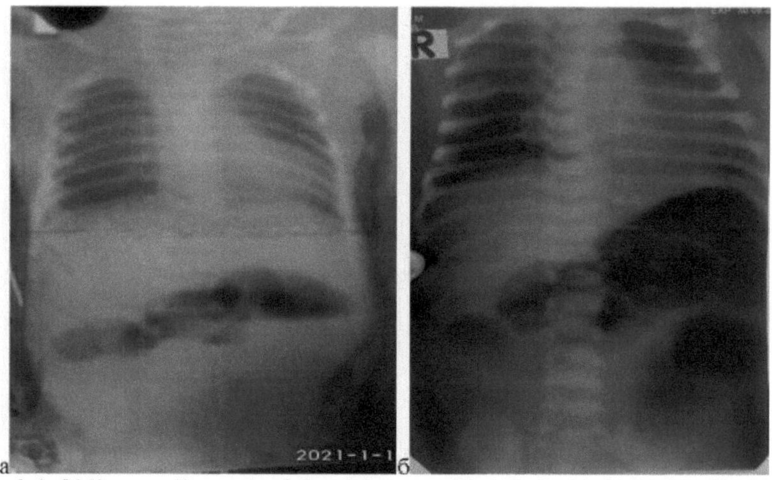

Fig.3.4. Oblique radiograph of the abdomen with ATnC: (a) Child S.F. I/B.#432 with distal atresia;
b) Child: K.S. I/B #443 with distal atresia

The diagnosis of UTI was suspected at ultrasound in 39 (34.5%) newborns. In 64 (56.6%), the diagnosis of CTCN caused difficulties due to partial low intestinal obstruction and cases of late hospitalisation of the child in a surgical hospital. To clarify the diagnosis, to detect congenital malformations of the colon and to determine the patency of the large intestine, X-ray contrast studies of the GI tract - irrigography (triombrast 76%) were performed in 24 (21.2%) cases, and GI tract passage - in 3 (2.6%). During irrigography 5-10 ml of contrast was injected. Irrigogram in VTCN allows differentiating ATNK, meconium ileus and Hirschprung's disease. The contrast agent is injected into the large intestine to avoid perforation due to mucus accumulation. If the contrast agent escapes under pressure without entering the bowel, a thorough revision of the large intestine is performed during surgery, taking into account the obstruction (Fig. 3.5.).

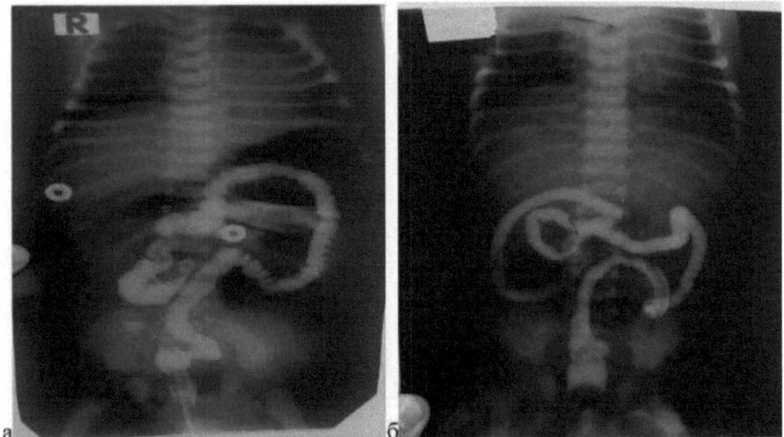

Fig.3.5.Irrigogram: a - b) patient M.Ch. I/B #147 and I.S. I/B #220 colon filled with contrast agent

The analysis of the obtained data showed that the leading methods in the diagnosis of VTCN are carefully collected maternal history, data of clinical and radiological methods of investigation. Fetal ultrasound is of high value in the diagnosis of this pathology. Radiological method as an additional method of investigation also has a special role due to the high percentage of cases of untimely diagnosis in congenital SCCI.

The causes of diagnostic errors are insufficient knowledge of the peculiarities of the clinical picture of the disease, errors in diagnosis, condensed clinical manifestations in patients with concomitant pathology and the presence of other malformations.

2.2. Results of laboratory and instrumental methods of examination of neonates with EIA on admission.

Table 3.1 shows the main laboratory values of neonates with VTCN at the time of hospitalisation.

Table 3.1.

Characteristics of laboratory parameters of newborns with VTCN at the time of hospitalisation in RCHS, (n=113)

Indicator	Results ш±5
Haemoglobin, g/l	170,3±25,4
Erythrocytes, 10 \L[12]	5,3±0,52
White blood cells, 10 \L[9]	11,7±4,49
Haematocrit, %	57,5±7,6
Total protein, gr/l	60,6±5,7
Urea, mmol/l	6,8±2,9
Total bilirubin, μm \L	99,4±44,5

C reactive protein, mg%	17,3±8,3
Glucose, mmol/L	3,2±2,2

When analysing the results of laboratory investigations, 23 (20.3%) children were confirmed to have IUI (leukocytosis, increased level of C-reactive protein) and systemic inflammatory response syndrome (SIRS).

Forty-eight (42.4%) newborns had high Hb, Ht and urea levels on admission due to weight loss and I-II degree exicosis. Children were often admitted to RCHC on the 2-3 day of life, and infusion therapy in maternity hospitals was inadequate relative to physiological needs or was not performed at all, which was due to late diagnosis and errors in management tactics.

An important factor in the development of multiorgan failure syndrome in neonates with VTCN is hypoglycaemia. Hypoglycaemia may not always be recognised if the diagnosis was based on clinical findings alone. Twenty-eight (24.7%) newborns had hypoglycaemia (below 2.2 mmol/l) on admission, confirming inadequate infusion therapy before and during interhospital transport of neonates with SCCN.

Studies of the haemostasis system showed that in 21 (18.5%) newborns with VTCN laboratory determined hypocoagulation due to PTI and thrombin test, moderate thrombocytopenia with normal or high levels of fibrinogen. This confirms that haemostasis disorders accompanied moderate hypocoagulation of the laboratory stage of acute DIC. The results of the haemostasis system in neonates with VTCN are presented in Table 3.2.

Table 3.2.

Indicators of haemostasis system of newborns with VTCN at the time of hospitalisation in RCHC (n=113)

Indicator	**Results** sh±5
Platelets, 10 \L^{9}	261±25,1
Fibrinogen A, gr/l	4,1±1,3
Prothrombin index, %	83,1±6,9
Thrombin test, st	3,14±0,9

On admission, newborns were performed the following: Ultrasound of internal organs, echocardiography (ECHO), neurosonography (NSG), to detect combined malformations and disorders of vital organs.

The nature of concomitant pathology is of great importance for the choice of treatment tactics in patients with jejunoileal atresia. In our practice, 36 (31.8%) newborns were diagnosed with various combinations of organ and system defects.

Table 3.3.

Newborns with multiple malformations (MMD) (n=113)

Types of malformations	**Number of patients**	
	abs	**%**
Cardiovascular malformations	21	18,5%

Malformations of the visual system	1	0,88%
Genitourinary malformations	12	10,6%
Musculoskeletal malformations	2	1,76%
Total	**36**	**31,8%**

Table 3.4.

Division of malformations in newborns with EIA(and=36)

Developmental defects	Quantity	
	abs	**%**
Heart and vascular malformations15 (47.7%)		
LTD.	9	25%
OAP	3	8,3%
VSD	1	2,7%
BFH	2	5,4%
Genitourinary malformations18 (50%)		
Congenital hydronephrosis	14	38,8%
Kidney agenesis	2	5,6%
Hypoplasia of the kidney	1	2,7%
Cryptorchidism	1	2,7%
Musculoskeletal malformations2 (5.4%)		
Incompleteness of the upper lip and palate	1	2,7%
clubfoot	1	2,7%
Visual system malformations1 (2.7%)		
Congenital retinal angiospasm	1	2,7%
Total	**36**	**100%**

Tables 3.4 and 3.5 present the variants of malformations we observed in neonates with VTCN. Thirty-six newborns with MVPD had defects of the MHS (50%), and of the SSS (47.7%). Analyses of each malformation in neonates with SCCN are presented in Table 3.6.

Table 3.6

Associated pathologies and complications in neonates with eunoileal atresia(n=113)

Nosology	Number of patients (n=113)	
	abs.	**frequency, %**
Congenital aspiration bronchopneumonia	113	100%
DIC	14	12,3%
Perinatal CNS damage	68	60,1%
Scleroma	5	4,42%
Hyperbilirubinaemia	27	23,9%

Anaemia	18	15,9%
Perforative peritonitis	23	20,3%
Severe sepsis	5	4,42%
Excysticosis	22	19,4%

The main number of associated pathologies and complications (DIC syndrome, scleroma, anaemia, perforative peritonitis, sepsis, excitosis) were the result of late diagnosis and inadequate tactics of patient management in maternity hospitals and during transport. Currently, the rates of all complications have decreased as a result of the introduction of methodological and tactical approaches to the diagnosis and management of patients with VTE at the prehospital stage.

The following complications were observed in EIA neonates: aspiration bronchopneumonia in 36 (31.8%) cases; respiratory failure (RF) in 45 (39.8%), hypovolemia in 22 (19.5%); body weight deficit from 2.5 to 27.6% in 28 (24.8%) cases, respectively. DIC was observed in 18 (16%) neonates, IUI in 23 (20.3%).

2.3. Measures to improve ante- and postnatal diagnosis and management tactics for neonates with childhood VTCN.

One of the strategies of the State social policy of our Republic is to strengthen the health of the population, in particular the health of mothers and children, to provide conditions for the birth and upbringing of healthy generations, to ensure early diagnosis of abnormalities in pregnancy and the development of newborns, to reduce the number of childhood disabilities, and to increase the competence of medical personnel in maternal and child health care.

The initiative has political and financial support from governments and organisations including WHO, UNICEF, UNFPA, World Bank.

As part of the consistent implementation of State programmes in the area of maternal and child health promotion and professional development of medical workers, the project "Effective Perinatal Care" was developed on the basis of analysis of the results of diagnosis and treatment of patients with CHD. International trainers were invited to implement this project at the initial stage. Seminars on the early detection, treatment and care of newborns were held at the Republican Perinatal Centre to improve the qualifications of neonatologists, anaesthesiologists-resuscitators, paediatric surgeons and obstetricians-gynaecologists and to train national trainers. Taking into account the shortage of personnel, the next step is to organise multiple field seminars and monitoring in the regions of the country.

As part of the implementation of State programmes, the Republican Training and Methodological Centre for Neonatal Surgery at the RTC was established on the basis of the neonatal surgery department of the RTC, and a course on "Neonatal surgery, anaesthesiology and resuscitation" was organised for the retraining of paediatric surgeons, anaesthesiologists and resuscitators. This became the educational and methodological basis for improving the treatment of children with VTCN.

Based on the results of these studies, we developed an algorithm for prenatal diagnosis and management of fetal VTE (Fig. 3.6) and an algorithm for postnatal diagnosis and management of newborns with VTE (Fig. 3.7).

Many years of experience in prenatal, early postnatal diagnosis allowed us to develop and propose an optimal scheme of invasive prenatal diagnosis and tactics for fetal ATnC (Fig.3.6) and (3.7).

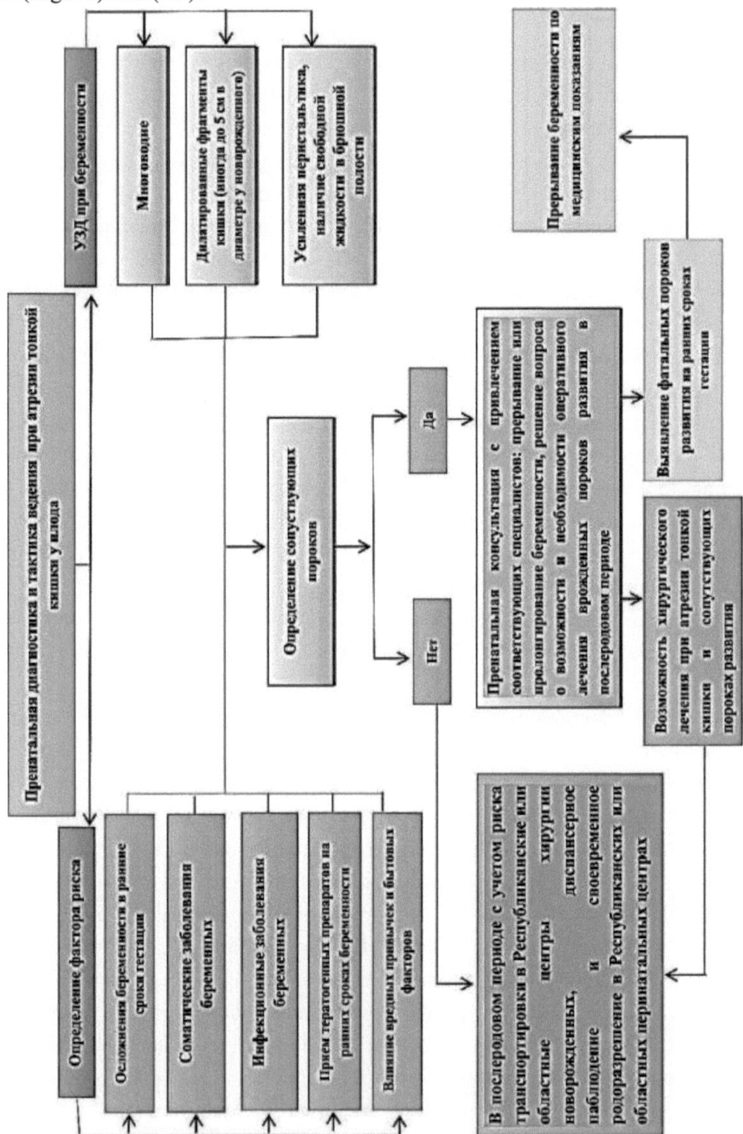

Figure 3.6. Algorithm of prenatal diagnostics and tactics for foetal EIA

This algorithm is based on commonly available methods of investigation, its application will help the surgeon to make the correct diagnosis in the shortest possible time and determine the treatment tactics.

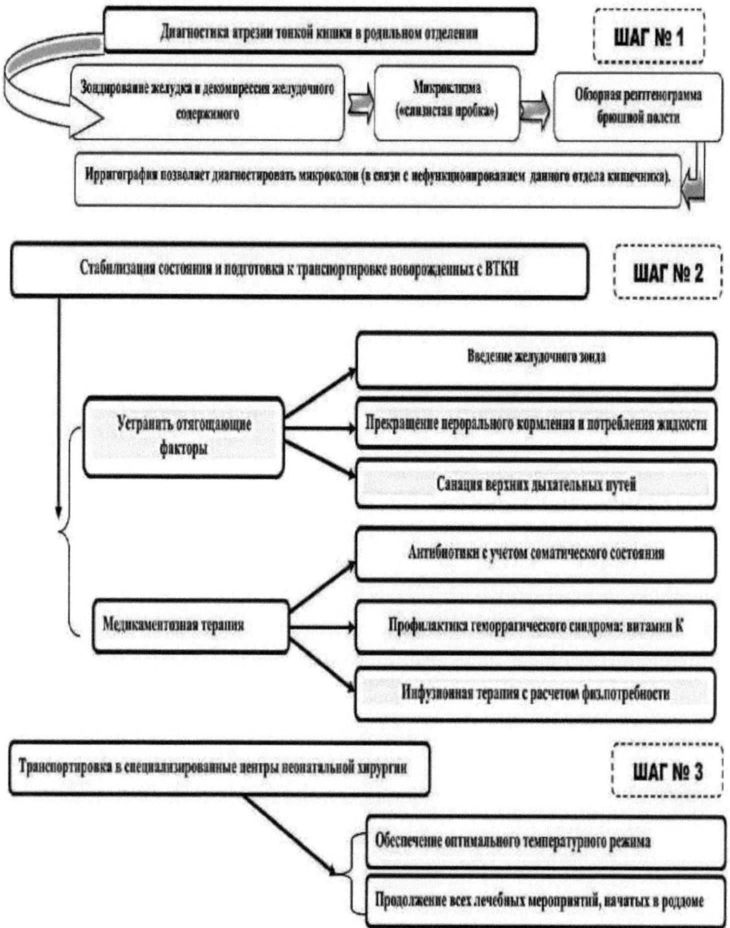

Figure 3.7. Algorithm of management of neonates with EIA

These algorithms (Fig. 3.6 and Fig. 3.7) represent all steps of early postnatal diagnosis and tactics of management of newborns with VTCN at the maternity hospital stage. Their application allowed to improve treatment results, reduce the incidence of complications and mortality (Conclusion on implementation of M3 RUz #8n-r/1319 dated 23.11.2022).

2.4. Results of prenatal diagnosis and assessment of clinical and anamnestic data of mothers of newborns with VTCN.

All (n=113) newborns admitted with EIA between 2014 and 2021 were analysed (Fig.3.1.): maternal health, social, obstetric and somatic status, course of the given pregnancy and labour, data of antenatal screening examinations, fetal-maternal factors and maternal age were assessed. We also analysed the clinical and functional data, anamnesis of the newborn, assessed the tactics of management in maternity institutions and the specifics of transport, and the results of diagnostic tests (Fig. 3.8).

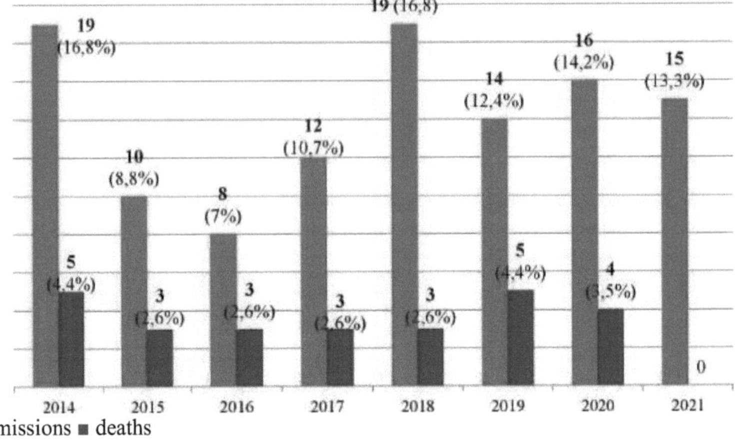

Figure 3.8: Enrolment of children with ENA from 2014 to 2021

2.4.1. Results of prenatal diagnosis and assessment of clinical and anamnestic data of mothers of newborns with VTCN

Antenatal diagnosis of EIA is based on such signs as polyhydroamnion (polyhydroamnion), dilated loops of the small intestine. The timing of patients' admission is presented in Table 3.7.

Table 3.7.

Timing of admission of patients to the RCHC with VTCN

Timing of patient admission (hours)	0-24	24-48	48-72	72 and more
Number of newborns admitted within this time frame	83 (73,5%)	22 (19,5%)	4 (3,5%)	4 (3,5%)

The data in the table show that 73.5% of patients with congenital small intestinal obstruction were hospitalised for the first 24 hours, 19.5% for the first two days, 3.5% for up to three days, and 3.5% of newborns were admitted more than three days after birth. Apparently, three main reasons influence late hospitalisation. One of them is that the diagnosis was not established in the antenatal period or the pregnant woman did not receive a full set of examinations.

The second reason is underestimation of clinical manifestations of congenital intestinal obstruction by medical personnel at the pre-hospital stage. Usually doctors refer to insufficient equipment of medical centres.

The third reason is the non-transportable state of the newborn or lack of transport. All these reasons have a negative impact on the prognosis of the disease, as patients are admitted to hospital with serious complications due to congenital intestinal disease with an obstruction.

The results of antenatal diagnosis are presented in Table 3.8.

Table 3.8.

Results of antenatal detection of fetal EIA (n=113)

	Antenatally diagnosed		**Suspicion of E.I.A.**		**Antenatally undiagnosed**		**Total number of**	
	abs	%	abs	%	abs	%	abs	%
In the context of the ROC.	28	24,7	9	7,9	-	-	37	32,7
In other institutions	11	9,7	2	1,7	63	55,7	76	67,3
Total	39	34,4	11	9,6	63	55,7	113	100

As can be seen from the table, out of 113 newborns37 (32.7%) were born in the Republican Perinatal Centre, 76 (67.3%) were admitted from other institutions. In 50 (44.2%) cases, the diagnosis was established in the foetus.

Obstruction and dilatation of fetal small bowel loops indicate the degree and level of intestinal obstruction. Increased fluid volume, multiple dilated small bowel loops, especially with hyperperistalsis and meconium particles in the lumen are the basis for the diagnosis of ATNK.

Prenatal diagnosis of small bowel obstruction is made at the turn of the second and third trimesters of gestation (Fig. 3.9).

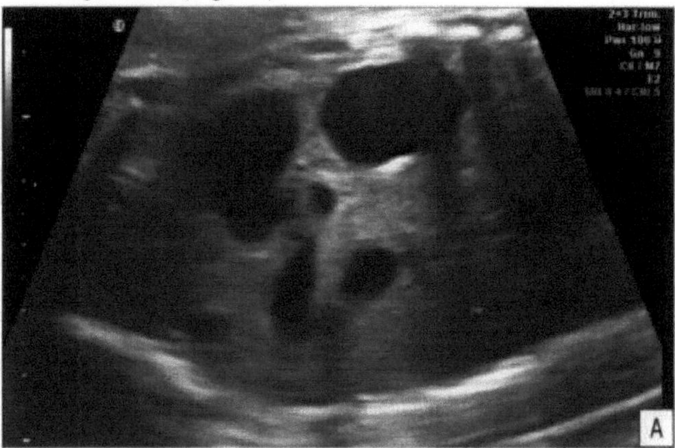

Figure 3.9 Fetal ultrasound with ATnC: no visualisation of the fetal stomach combined with polyuria, pregnant woman A.D. I/B No. 1038

Of the 50 children with antenatally diagnosed ICH, 28 (56%) had CTCI detected at the RTC where prenatal counselling was done with the participation of concerned specialists. These pregnant women were registered at the ROC and were followed up by obstetrician-gynaecologist and neonatal surgeon. In 11 (9.7%) cases, the diagnosis of fetal SCCN was made in other institutions, and these women were also referred to the RTC for further follow-up.

A total of 11 (9.7%) cases had suspected fetal SCCN in the antenatal period. Of the 9 children born in RTCs, antenatal suspicion of SCCN was registered in 7 (6.2%). Among those admitted from other health facilities, suspicion occurred in 1.76% of cases. Antenatally, the diagnosis was not established in 63 (54%) children admitted from other institutions.

Antenatal fetal ultrasound revealed multiple congenital malformations in 36 (31.8%) of 113 pregnant women. In the structure of fetal MCDD, 11 (9.7%) had congenital malformations of the urinary system (11 (9.7%)); 21 (18.6%) had cardiovascular malformations (CHD, FVHD); and 4 (3.5%) had musculoskeletal and other malformations;

Fetal ATCN was diagnosed at 24 to 28 weeks of gestation, and the minimum time for ATC diagnosis was 25 to 26 weeks. In all patients at prenatal diagnosis of ATC in the third trimester of gestation, the intestinal loops were dilated up to 15 mm. In the second trimester of gestation, small bowel obstruction was first suspected when its transverse size exceeded 7 mm, increased peristalsis and meconium particles in the lumen.

We analysed the course of antenatal and intrapartum periods based on the history of the studied children with EIA.

The age gradation showed that children with EIA were born to mothers aged between 18 and 39 years, the mean age was 25.8±4.85 years (Table 3.3).

It should be emphasised that 21 (18.6%) babies were born by caesarean section, of which 7 (33.4%) were born between 30 and 35 weeks of gestation. In 7 (33.4%) of these cases, the indication for caesarean section was multigestationalism, and in 2 (9.5%) cases, fetal ICH. Although fetal ICH itself was not a direct indication for operative delivery, it had a negative impact on treatment outcomes. There were 28 (24.7%) first-time mothers and 85 (75.3%) repeat mothers (Table 3.8).

Table 3.8.

Age characteristics of mothers of newborns with EIA (n=113)

Mother's age	Number (n=113)	
	abs.	%
18-25 years old	46	40,7%
26-35 years old	37	32,8%
35 years and older	30	26,5%
Total	113	100%

The most common unfavourable factors affecting pregnant women in early pregnancy were: acute respiratory viral infection (ARVI) in some cases with hyperthermia, which was observed in 104 (92%) pregnant women. The high prevalence of viral infections in the patients was due to the fact that their pregnancies predominantly occurred at the time of the highest prevalence of acute respiratory viral infections.

TORCH-infection with a pronounced pathogenic property was noted in 21 (18.5%) cases. Bacterial infection in the form of acute and chronic extragenital foci (pyelonephritis, parotitis, stomatitis, acute respiratory infections, rheumatism, phlegmon) was detected in 12 (10.6%) women, genital colpitis in 3 (2.6%).

Among the somatic pathologies that can influence the formation of fetal EIA, anaemia was more common in 61 (54%) pregnant women; cardiac pathology in 7 (6.2%); and thyroid pathology in 21 (18.6%).

Administration of drugs in early pregnancy (antibiotics of various groups, non-steroidal anti-inflammatory drugs; antithyroids) could have teratogenic effects and lead to the development of VTCN in 86 (76%) cases. Exposure to nicotine through "passive smoking" was found in 47 (41.6%) women, pregnant smokers constituted 3.5%. Contact with pesticides was found in 8 (7%) women. 64 (56.6%) women had a history of multiple pregnancy.

Thus, the identified features of the course of pregnancy in fetal women may serve as clinical markers of fetal VTCN, as seen in the diagram (Fig.3.10.).

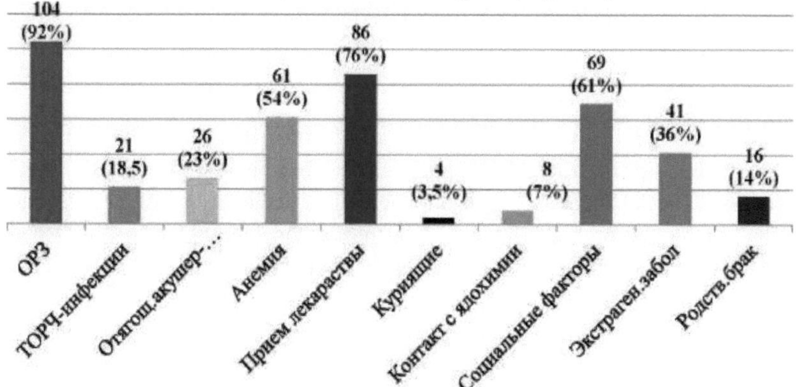

Figure 3.10.Risk factors in early pregnancy that may serve as clinical markers in the prenatal diagnosis of fetal SCCN

Based on our analysis, we concluded that in addition to the triad of signs (multivagina, multiple dilated small bowel loops, increased peristalsis with floating meconium particles), risk factors for the birth of children with VTCN are of great importance.

The most significant factors are the following:

- threatened abortion;
- somatic and infectious diseases of the woman during pregnancy;
- exposure to medication;
- exposure to environmental factors.

Early admission of patients to a specialised hospital is of great importance for a favourable outcome of the disease. Figure 3.11 shows the timing of children's admission to hospital (24 hours from birth).

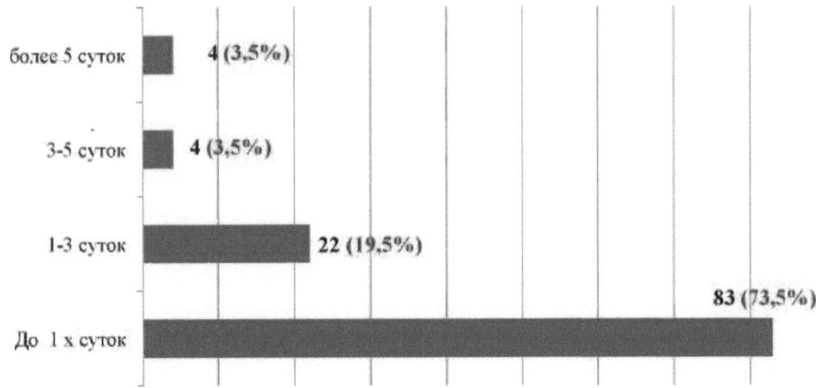

Fig. 3.11. Timing of children's admission to RCHS

As shown in Figure 3.4, newborns were hospitalised in the first 24 hours of life in 73.5%, 1-3 days in 19.5%, and later in 7% of cases respectively, indicating poor early diagnosis of VTCN in maternity hospitals.

The table (Table 3.4) presents the clinical and anamnestic status of newborns with VTCN on admission to the RCHC. When assessing the clinical and anamnestic data of the newborn, special attention was paid to the time of diagnosis in the postnatal period (before or after feeding); the nature of diagnostic and therapeutic measures before admission to our clinic and the severity of the condition on admission.

The results of the study showed that in 50 (44.2%) of the cases, neonates were diagnosed with VTCN after feeding, i.e. they were put to the breast after birth, which was the cause of aspiration pneumonia, taking into account the fact that in 7 of them there was a suspicion of VTCN due to polyuria. Inadequate therapeutic interventions due to late diagnosis of severe exicosis were observed in 14 (12.3%) newborns (Table 3.9).

Table 3.9

Clinical and anamnestic status of newborns (n=113)

Indicators		**Total number(n=113)**	
		abs.	**%**
Put to the breast (breastfed)	Yes	50	44,2
	No	63	55,8
Stabilisation of the newborn before transport	Adequately	48	42,5
	Inadequate	22	19,4
	Not conducted	**43**	**38,1**
Body temperature	**Hypothermia**	**21**	**18,6**
	Norma	84	74,3
	Hyperthermia	8	7,1
Presence of severe exicosis	Got it	14	12,3
	No	99	87,7

The presence of a stomach tube	Got it	79	70
	No	**34**	**30**
Therapeutic measures during transport	Held	107	95
	None	**6**	**5**
Respiratory failure	It didn't manifest itself	68	60,1
	I-II degree	42	37,2
	III degree	3	2,7
Severity of condition of a newborn on admission	Heavy	81	71,7
	Very heavy	23	20,4
	Extremely difficult	9	7,9

2.5. Analysis of hospitalised neonates with VTCN

Requirements for preparation of newborns for transportation to a specialised hospital are based on anatomo-physiological nuances and urgency of the formed GI pathology, so it is necessary to observe the temperature regime (transport incubator is recommended), to control oxygenation by pulse oximeters and transcutaneous sensors (changes in constants have a detrimental effect on newborns), to maintain a constant glycaemic level, as newborns have minimal glycogen reserves with high energy demand (prevention of hypoglycaemia),

In our study 77 (68%) neonates were transported with gross malpractices. This led to hypothermia in 21 (18.6%) neonates and severe hypoglycaemia in 28 (24.7%).

Timely diagnosis of VTCN and proper preparation in maternity hospitals before transport was observed in 53(47%) cases, inadequate primary stabilisation in 51(45%), the above measures were not performed at all in 9(8%) cases.

Another factor ensuring the safety of interhospital transport is compliance with the basic principle of resuscitation and consultative teams' activity - threatometry, predicting the degree of risk and the immediate outcome of transport. 16(14.1%) patients were admitted by gravity without the accompaniment of medical personnel, which led to the deterioration of the newborn's condition due to non-compliance with the rules of transport.

An important aspect of interhospital transport of newborns in critical condition is the continuation of intensive care, ensuring its continuity at all stages of the treatment process. During transport, all therapeutic measures initiated in Level 1 and II hospitals or at the stage of preparation of the child for transport should be carried out.

The results of the study showed that in43 (38%) cases the rules of interhospital transport were violated: the newborns were not given the necessary therapeutic measures, which led to destabilisation of the newborns' condition.

Virtually any critical condition in the newborn period may be accompanied by significant impairment of gas exchange and oxygenation, which requires the organisation of respiratory support during transport. Given the anatomical and pathogenetic features of this malformation, it is necessary to minimise this risk.

34 (30%) children were transported without oro-ili nasogastric tube and aspiration of gastric contents, leading to complications of respiratory failure of varying severity.

It is known that newborn babies have a pronounced immaturity of thermoregulation mechanisms, which favours heat loss by infrared radiation. The need for oxygen in a hypothermic child can increase three or more times! More often hypothermia occurs in critical conditions such as asphyxia in labour, respiratory failure, sepsis and other negative consequences. In addition to hypoxia, acidosis, respiratory depression, apnoea, depression of consciousness and seizures are observed.

Analysis of the data showed that due to violation of the rules of transport and management of neonates with VTCN, patients were admitted in hypothermia (<36.0°C) in 21 (18.6%); in hyperthermia (>37.5°C)in 8 (7%) cases, respectively.

Thus, for a number of reasons: violations in screening diagnosis, obstetric tactics, delayed diagnosis and, as a consequence, late transfer to a specialised hospital, violation of transport rules, all this led to the fact that 20.4% of newborns were delivered in a very serious condition, 7.9% were delivered in a very serious condition. All this had a negative impact on the course of the disease and required longer preoperative preparation.

Based on our analysis, we concluded that during the preparation of the child for and during transport, all efforts should be directed at preventing the four most significant pathological conditions, any of which may provoke the development of a syndrome of multiple organ dysfunction and failure against the background of already existing VTCN (Fig. 3.12.).

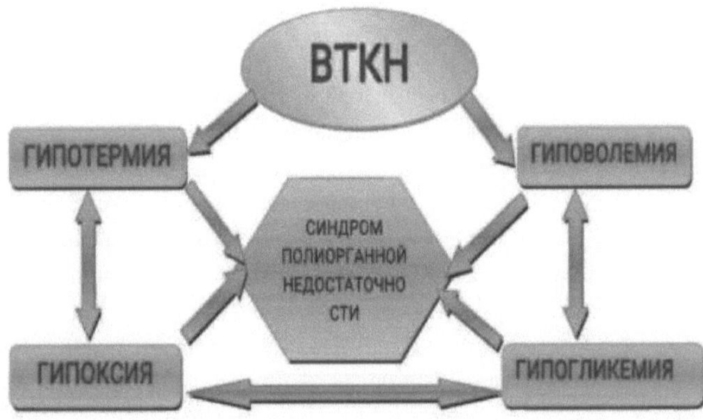

Figure 3.12: Major risk factors aggravating the condition of a neonate with SCCN at the stage of interhospital transport.

Summary of the chapter

The results of EIA diagnosis in newborns from 2014 to 2021 showed that the severity of the condition of newborns with VTCN on admission was due to various

complications and the development of multi-organ failure syndrome on the background of VTCN due to late diagnosis and incorrect management tactics in these patients.
The share of antenatal diagnosis of SCCN in the country is currently 6.3%. This is a critically low percentage of screening examinations performed on pregnant women, which does not allow to identify ultrasound signs of VTE in the foetus to the necessary extent.
When analysing the peculiarities of the course of pregnancy in women with fetal SCCN, it has been proved that the identification of risk factors early in pregnancy increases the chances of identifying the anomaly, and the risk factors themselves can serve as clinical markers in the prenatal diagnosis of fetal SCCN. The following factors accounted for the highest percentage: threat of abortion (68%), acute respiratory infections (92%), TORCH infection (18.5%), anaemia (54%), and drug exposure (76%).
Our studies have shown that timely postnatal diagnosis and adequate preparation of newborns with VTCN for transport in maternity hospitals was carried out only in 53 (47%) patients. 51 (45%) newborns were inadequately treated in maternity hospitals, and 9 (7.9%) children were not treated at all. 77 (68%) newborns were transported with gross violations of the rules, resulting in hypothermia in 21 (18.6%) cases and severe hypoglycaemia in 28 (24.7%). When preparing a child for and during transport, all efforts should be directed at preventing the four most important pathological conditions: hypothermia, hypoxia, hypovolaemia, and hypoglycaemia. Any of them can provoke the development of multiorgan dysfunction syndrome and failure on the background of VTCN.
Thus, the results of ante- and postnatal diagnosis allowed us to develop and implement algorithms for pre- and postnatal diagnosis and management of patients with VTCN. Their application helps to reduce the incidence of complications and mortality in the pre- and postoperative periods.

CHAPTER IV

ANALYSING THE RESULTS OF SURGICAL TREATMENT.

4.1 Selection of treatment method and determination of the scope of surgical intervention in neonates

Surgical correction for neovaginal neovaginal disease was performed on 1.6±0.55 days of life after stabilisation of the child's condition and completion of all necessary diagnostic measures. The choice of the volume of surgery was made individually, depending on the course of the pathological process, the level of atresia and morphological changes in the intestinal tube.

The history of surgical treatment of newborns with jejunoileal atresia in the RCHS was conventionally divided into 2 stages.

First stage of EIA treatment at the RCHS: 2014-2017.

At the initial stage of our work, we had an emergency operation, which consisted of primary anastomosis or enterostomy using traditional methods. This was a somewhat erroneous tactic, but at that time it was the only possibility to save the life of the newborn.

The analysis of mortality showed that the most common causes of death were causes of septic and haemorrhagic genesis due to late diagnosis and surgical postoperative complications. Often patients at the time of hospitalisation had edema-haemorrhagic and DIC, aggravated by surgical intervention and in the postoperative period.

By the end of the first stage we managed to reduce postoperative mortality from27% to 13.5% (2 times). Among the causes of death in 26 children were postoperative non-surgical complications: general and specific. At stage 1, we needed to minimise postoperative complications as much as possible and preserve the life of the newborn. However, the increasing flow of patients with severe comorbidities due to late diagnosis and incorrect management tactics did not improve the situation.

Phase II treatment of a newborn with EIA at the RCHS: 2017-2021.

In 2017-2021, the challenges became very apparent, without addressing them, it was difficult to achieve a positive outcome.

Firstly, the problems of late diagnosis and inadequate management of neonates with EIA at the maternity hospital stage became acute, which in most cases led to an unfavourable outcome. In peripheral institutions, the opinion among physicians about ATNK as a fatal malformation persisted. Many of them did not maintain clinical protocols on the diagnosis and management of patients with this malformation.

Secondly, the relatively high incidence of suture failure during intestinal anastomosis (if the surgeon does not take into account the ratio of the diameter of the driving and withdrawing intestine when applying the interintestinal anastomosis) in the traditional way caused the development of peritonitis with lethal outcome.

All of the above made us reconsider some of the established views on the problem of surgical correction of EIA.

We compared the two methods of surgical treatment and divided the patients into two groups. The main group included 37(33%) children (video-assisted route) and the control group included 76(67%) children (traditional route). In our institutions, we started to operate on children using video-assisted route from the end of 2017 (Fig.4.1.)

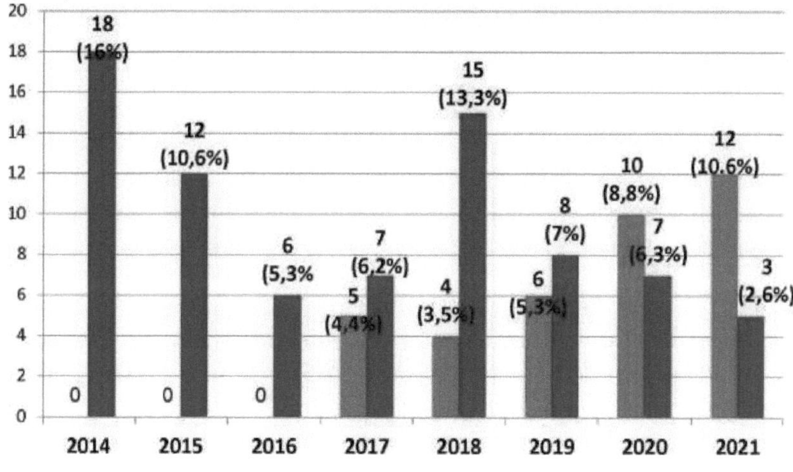

■ Main group ■ Control group

Fig.4.1.Ratio and distribution of patients by the method of surgery (n=113)

Patients were divided into two groups to compare the efficacy of surgical techniques.

Main group - 37 (33%) patients who underwent video-assisted laporoscopic revision of abdominal cavity organs; minilaparotomy; mobilisation of the atresized small intestine and excretion through a minilaparotomy incision.

Control - 76 (67%) neonates who underwent laparotomy; revision of abdominal cavity organs.

Preoperative preparation. Newborns with ATK and AIC were given standard preoperative preparation: "adequate compensation of fluid and electrolyte losses, warming, sugar control, decompression of the upper GI tract with mandatory consideration of the volume of losses" [49]. [49].

In case of ATNK in the initial segment, for effective decompression of the blind segment of the jejunum there is a need for a gastric tube, in such cases preoperative preparation is delayed for 1-2 days to normalise homeostasis. In neonatal ATNK it is necessary to perform surgical correction for the first day of life to prevent ischaemia and perforation of the driving segment.

In cases of severe flatulence, preoperative artificial ventilation should be performed in some cases.

Preoperative preparation was carried out for an average of 16.3±9.9 hours during the first observation period and 14.2±9.8 hours during the second. Preoperative infusion therapy - glucose solution in the volume of age-specific fluid requirements (10% glucose solution with saline). Volaemic drugs were administered in the second one in

4 (5%) cases.

All patients were prescribed antibacterial, haemostatic therapy before surgical intervention: received newborns of the first and second study group.

The criteria of adequacy of preoperative preparation were restoration of haemodynamics, water-electrolyte balance, optimal diuresis in both groups.

Preoperative preparation programme: respiratory support of patients with respiratory and/or cardiac failure, hypovolemic shock and impaired CSF. Infusion therapy of 10-20 ml/kg*hour with glucose-salt solutions, fresh frozen plasma, albumin was performed.

To improve microcirculation and correct haemodynamic disorders, inotropic support with dopamine at a dose of 2-5 mcg/kg*min was performed, sometimes - hormone therapy.

Vitamin K, dicinone, sodium ethamsylate, and tremin were used to prevent DIC and haemorrhage.

Antibiotic therapy implied cephalosporins of 2-3 generations + aminoglycosides + metranidazole.

Gastrointestinal decompression was performed with a gastric tube (Fr#6, if more than 3000 grams of weight then Fr#8) with lavage with physiological solution.

The following criteria were used to assess the effectiveness of preoperative preparation: "hemodynamic normalisation, normalisation of heart rate and BP, disappearance of the "white spot" symptom, acrocyanosis, skin marbling, normalisation of body temperature, appearance of diuresis, improvement of acid-base state".

Acute renal failure due to inadequate therapy before admission to the surgical hospital and aggravation of hypovolaemic shock was observed in 3 infants of the first group and 1 of the second group.

The **assessment of surgical stress levels** intraoperatively was based on: "the length of the incision on the anterior abdominal wall, duration of surgical intervention and anaesthesia, the amount of narcotic analgesics and myorelaxants consumed during surgery, the amount of blood loss, and the occurrence of complications". In the early postoperative period: "duration of stay in the intensive care and intensive care unit (ICU), number of bed days, severity of pain syndrome, restoration of intestinal peristalsis, initiation of enteral load, cosmetic effect, number of complications".

In conjunction with the literature, the supraumbilical transverse incision with good exposure of the intestine, but with a high risk of adhesions, was considered to be the most optimal. The advantages of these incisions are a low postoperative scar, low intensity of postoperative pain and a low proportion of intra-abdominal adhesions.

According to the traditional method under intubation anaesthesia, surgical intervention was started with a transverse incision (laparatomy) 5.5 - 6.5 cm above the umbilicus and revision of the abdominal cavity.

In the traditional method of surgery in the absence of inflammation and moderate dilatation of the driving loop of the small intestine, 36 (46.1%) patients underwent

direct anastomosis, including 5 (14%) patients with narrowing of the driving section, and 29 (80.5%) patients underwent "fish mouth" anastomosis ("fish mouth" by J.Louw).
(Figure 4.2.).

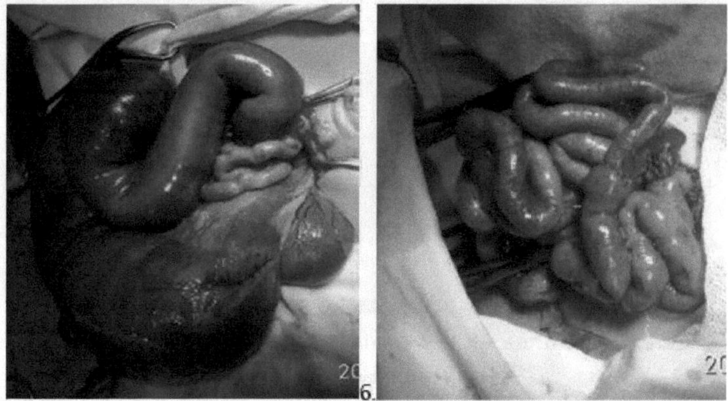

Fig.4.2 Patient A. (f.m.) I/B #373. Intraoperative picture in ileum atresia: (a) type II atresia before anastomosis;
b) final appearance of the fish-mouth end-to-end anastomosis

In most cases, ATNK is accompanied by a large difference in the diameter of the affected areas. The large difference in intestinal diameters made it impossible to apply an end-to-end anastomosis. In such conditions, we used end-to-side unloading anastomoses in 6 (12.8%) neonates (Fig. 4.3). 5 (10.6%) infants underwent membranotomy for type I atresia (Fig. 4.4.).

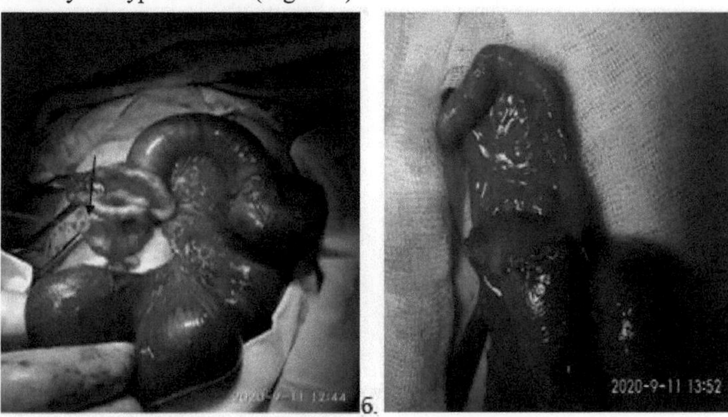

Fig.4.3 Patient F.M. (f.m.). I/B #752. Intraoperatively in ileum atresia: a) type III A atresia: "V"-shaped defect of the mesentery, total length of the small intestine within the normal range; the narrowed diverting intestine is indicated by the arrow; b) final view of the end-to-side anastomosis from the front.

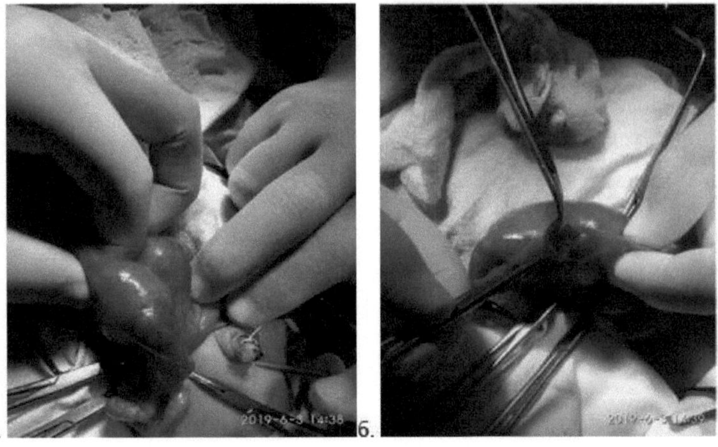

Fig.4.4 Patient E.V. (f.m.). I/B #526. Intraoperative picture of jejunal atresia: a) type I atresia;
b) condition after membranotomy

In case of high ATC location, a naso-gastro-intestinal (intubator) tube was maximally passed beyond the anastomosis zone in 10 (13%) patients. This resulted in temporary decompression of the small intestinal loop for a short time, restored peristalsis, prevented postoperative complications and anastomosis suture failure (Fig. 4.5).

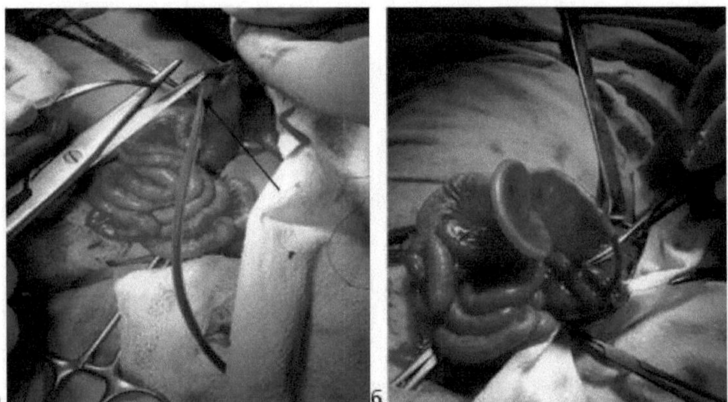

Fig.4.5. Patient M.N. (f.m.). I/B #1235. Intraoperative picture in jejunal atresia Ntip: a) intubator tube is indicated by an arrow. b) period of anastomosis application.

The mesenteric defect was sutured with separate knotted sutures. As much as possible, we did not leave the drainage in the abdominal cavity, because it is also considered a gateway for infection, fibroadhesive peritonitis. In 8(10.2%) cases we performed drainage of the abdominal cavity to ensure fluid outflow and timely diagnosis of anastomosis suture failure (partial and complete) and peritonitis. Then haemostasis was performed along the course of the operation. Layer-by-layer sutures were applied to the wound. Aseptic dressing (Fig. 4.6).

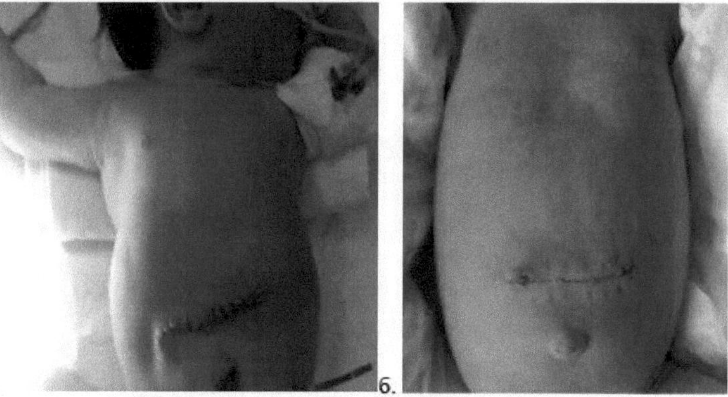

Fig. 4.6. Patient K. (f.m.) Postoperative transverse incision: a. anterior view; b. after suture removal on day 14.

In the postoperative period, secondary wound healing was observed in 7(8.9%) patients and anastomosis failure in 6(7.7%) patients.

For the first time, video-assisted neonatal surgery (VAS) for jejunoileal atresia was started at the RCHS at the end of 2017.

All BACs were performed according to the standard: ".... the first trocar was inserted to insert the laparoscope and revise the abdominal cavity, then the trocars were placed under the working instruments, partial mobilisation of the intestine was performed, the main vessels were treated, and the resection boundaries were set".

To perform BAC surgeries in our patients we used: "endosurgical complex (4K rack) with a set of equipment including a video camera with optical cable and 5 and 10 mm laparoscope, light source with light guide, monitor, insufflator with continuously adjustable modes of CO2 supply, system for aspiration of contents from the abdominal cavity, electrosurgical unit with modes of bi- and monopolar coagulation, high-frequency electrosurgical system "ERBE" with BiClamp instrument of 5 mm diameter, a set of trocars of 3 mm, 5 mm, 10 mm diameter and instruments of 3 and 5 mm".

Technique of video-assisted surgery. The child was placed on the operating table in the anti-Trendelenburg position with 30° rotation of the body to the left.

Under intubation anaesthesia, in the supine position, after treatment of the operating field in the infraumbilical area, the first trocar (2 mm in diameter) was placed, CO_2 was insufflated and pneumoperitoneum was created. Then we installed an optic with a 5 mm NORKKHYZP rod and under the control of the optic a trocar (3.0 mm) to the right of the umbilicus. Further, during revision of the abdominal cavity in case of adhesions, the adhesions were disconnected with a bipolar coagulator. The atresised part of the small intestine, the distal end, which looked like a "cord", was detected.

The presence of mesenteric defect was determined. Further, a minilararatomic incision from 2.0 cm to 3.0 cm was made at the trocar site on the right side and the atresised parts of the small intestine were withdrawn. The patency of the diverting end of the intestine was checked, and the atresised part of the small intestine was resected. At inter-intestinal manastomosis, the intestinal loops were carefully immersed into the abdominal cavity. The abdominal cavity was not drained as much as possible because it is also a gateway for infection. A double-barrel enterostomy was inserted through a minilaparatomic incision. Haemostasis in the course of the operation. Layer-by-layer wound sutures and aseptic dressing were applied. The figure (Fig. 4.7. from I to X) shows the sequence of video-assisted surgery.

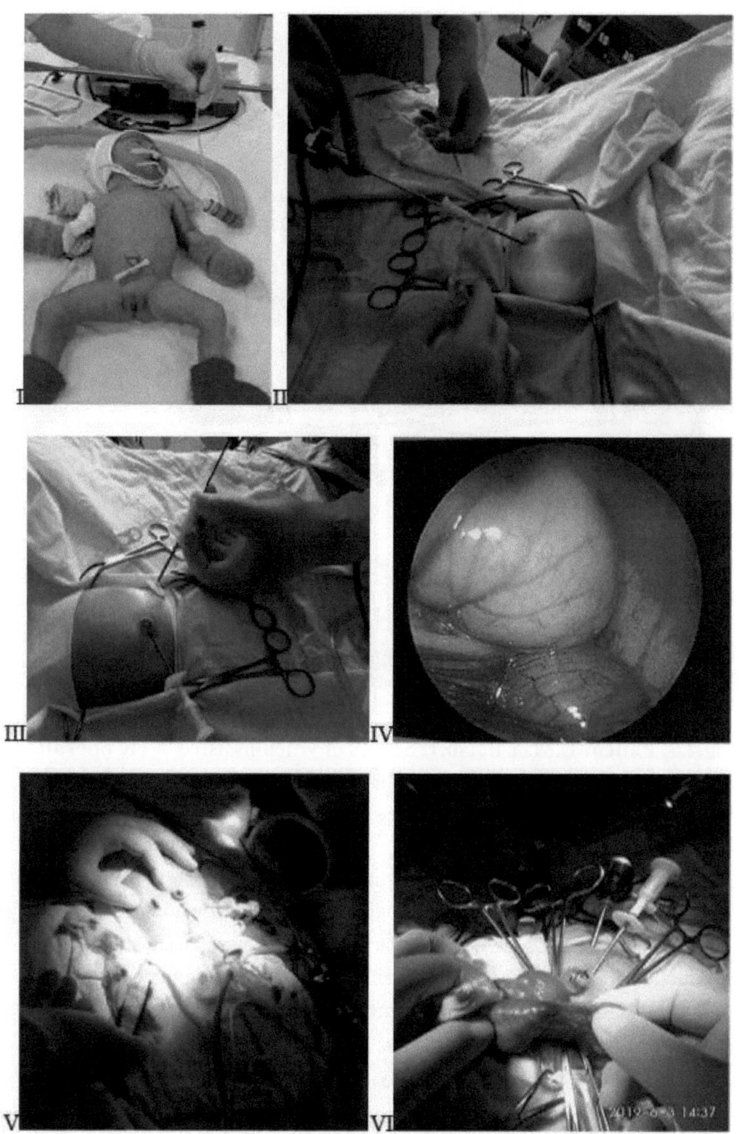
I
II
III
IV
V
VI

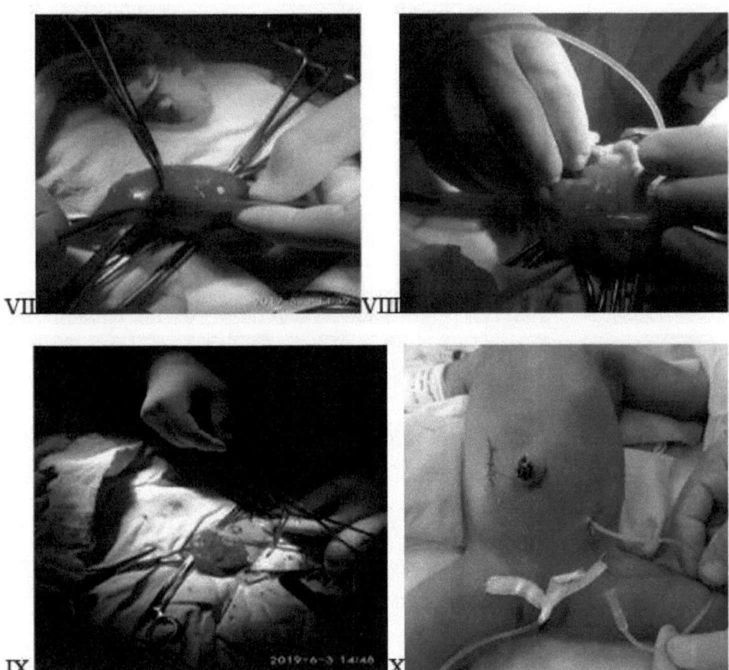

Fig.4.7. Patient E.M. I/B. No.1. Stages of video-assisted ATK operation.

The upper transverse incision for EIA surgery is based on the tenets of minimally invasive surgery and has better intra- and postoperative outcomes relative to transrectal access.

In the main group, 2 (5.7%) patients underwent transverse incision access and 26(74%) patients underwent transrectal incision access. In the control group, 32 (41%) transverse incisions and 12(15.3%) transrectal incisions were performed.

The introduction of minimally invasive techniques in the treatment of VTCN resulted in a minimal decrease in the incidence of fatal outcomes and postoperative complications.

BAC, according to the results of our study, is recognised as a better surgical treatment tactic for congenital neonatal ileal obstruction and should be performed in all possible cases of surgical interventions in neonates with superior results in the early postoperative period.

BAC has superior cosmetic results, results in minimal surgical trauma and a more favourable early postoperative course of patients with EIA (Fig.4.8).

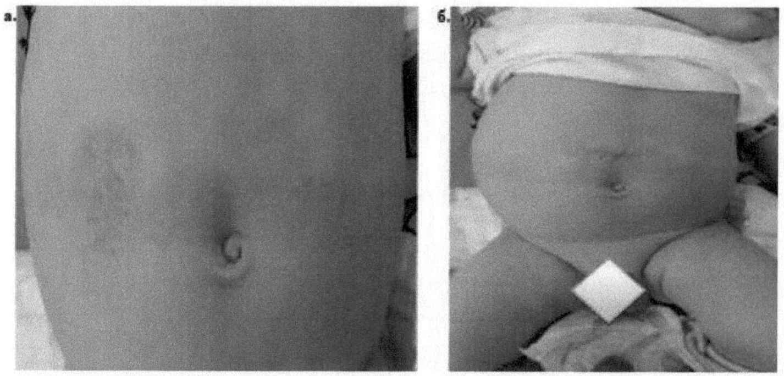

Fig.4.8. Catamnesis. Postoperative picture: a) patient R.S. (f.m.) I/B. No. 208. at transrectal incision, anterior view; b) patient E.M. I/B. No. 570 at transrectal incision, anterior view after suture removal.

With a large variety of clinical guidelines, protocols, and standards, a paediatric surgeon under time constraints needs a concise algorithm for surgical treatment of patients with EIA. We have developed an algorithm for operated patients with VTCN (Fig. 4.9.).

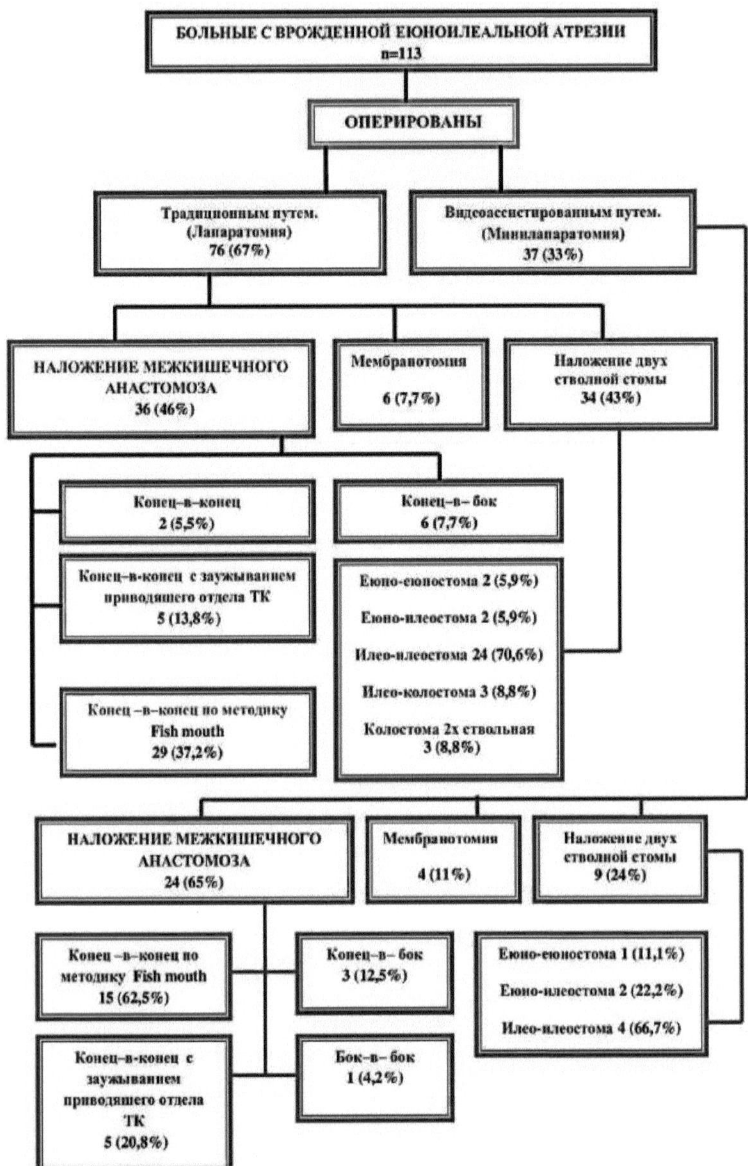

Fig. 4.9. Types of surgical interventions performed on children with ATNC

We have developed an algorithm of treatment and complex rehabilitation after surgical correction of ATK (Fig.4.10).

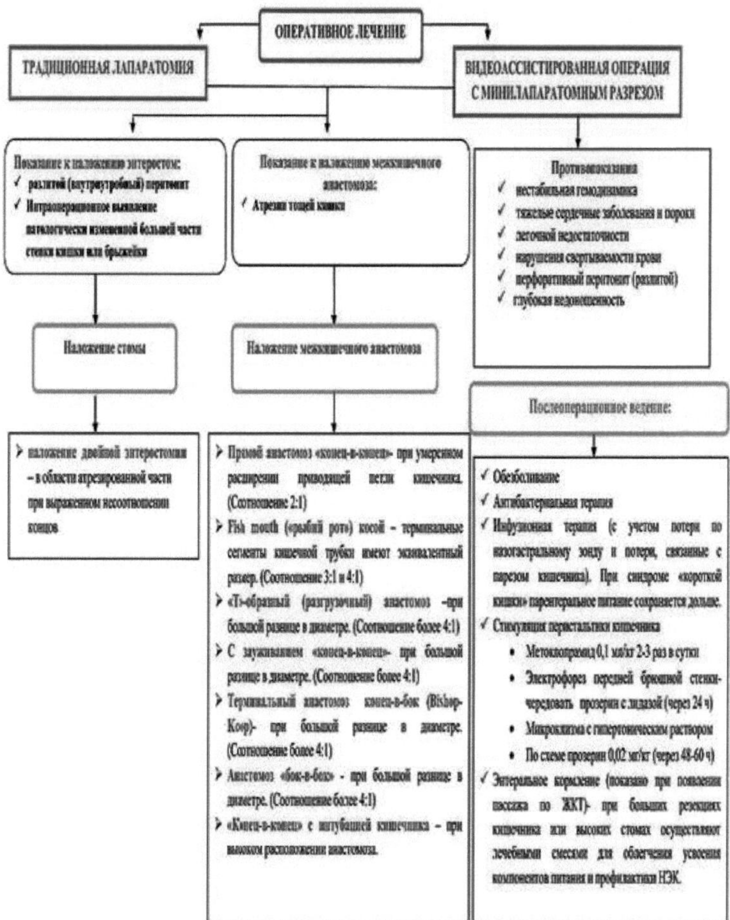

Fig.4.10. Algorithm of treatment and complex rehabilitation of children after surgical correction of ATNK

The data of our study allow us to consider video-assisted laparoscopy as a safe surgical approach in the treatment of obstructive congenital jejunoileal obstruction. At the same time in the postoperative period secondary wound healing was observed in 1 (2,8%) patient and anastomosis failure - in 2 (5,7%) children. The postoperative scar on the skin of the anterior abdominal wall was practically imperceptible.

After completion of the previous stage of surgery, all our patients underwent minilaparotomy with localisation of the incision to the anterior abdominal wall depending on the pathological focus. In children operated on by BAC, the size of the skin incision ranged from 2.5 to 4 cm (mean, 3.5±0.9 cm).

Table.4.1.

Volume of surgical intervention in the compared groups by type and parts of VTCN

TYPES	I		II		IIIa		IIIb		IV	
(n=113)	14 (12,5%)		23 (20,5%)		43 (38%)		20 (17,5%)		13 (11,5%)	
Atresised part	ATK	AGRO-INDUSTRIAL COMPLEX	ATK	AGRO-INDUSTRIAL COMPLEX	ATK	AGRO-INDUSTRIAL COMPLEX	ATK	AGRO-INDUSTRIAL COMPLEX	ATK	AGRO-INDUSTRIAL COMPLEX
Traditional 76(67%)	7 (51%)	2 (14%)	3 (13%)	10 (44%)	13 (30%)	21 (49%)	7 (35%)	9 (45%)	4 (31%)	1 (7,5%)
YOU 37(33%)	4 (28%)	1 (7%)	6 (26%)	4 (17%)	5 (12%)	4 (9%)	3 (15%)	1 (5%)	7 (54%)	1 (7,5%)
Total(n=113) (100%)	11 (79%)	3 (21%)	9 (39%)	14 (61%)	18 (42%)	25 (58%)	11 (50%)	9 (50%)	11 (85%)	1 (14%)

Note:* **ATK**- jejunal atresia, ***APK**- ileum atresia.

In the main group, 26 (70%) patients underwent surgery with interintestinal anastomosis, 7 (20%) - with double-barrel enterostomy. In47 (62%) patients of the control group the surgery ended with interintestinal anastomosis, in 31 (41%) patients - with double-barrel enterostomy. The results of VAM and traditional surgeries are shown in Table 4.1.

A comparative analysis of the operations performed and their number in the main and control groups is presented in Table 4.2.

Table 4.2.

Comparative analysis between the main group and the control group

groups Number of operations	**Main group (n=37)** 37	**Control group (n=76)** 76
Eunotomy	4	5
Resection of small intestine with euno-jejunoanastomosis with narrowing	5	4
Small bowel resection with end-to-end jejuno-jejunoanastomosis **(Fishmouth)**	8	6
Small intestine resection with side-to-side jejuno-jejunoanastomosis	1	-
Small intestine resection with end-to-side jejuno-jejunoanastomosis	-	3
Small bowel resection with end-to-end ileo-ileoanastomosis with narrowing **(Fishmouth)**	2	1
Small bowel resection with end-to-end ileo-ileoanastomosis **(Fishmouth)**	3	6
Small intestine resection with end-to-side	1	-

ileoanastomosis		
Small intestine resection with end-to-side ileo-ileoanastomosis	2	3
Small bowel resection with end-to-end ileo-ileoanastomosis **(Fishmouth)**	4	14
Small intestine resection with end-to-end colo-colonic anastomosis	-	2
Small intestine resection with end-to-end ileo-colonastomosis	-	3
Bivalve jejunostomy	1	2
Double-barrel eunoileostomy.	2	2
Bivalve ileostomy	4	24
Bivalve ileocolostomy	-	3
Bivalve colostomy	-	2

1.2 Comparative characteristics of the immediate and long-term results of surgical treatment of patients with EIA.

The absence of reliable difference between the main and control groups in terms of the volume and nature of operations makes it possible to objectively assess the results of treatment. The duration of operations in the main group was 90-290 minutes, on average 182±37.9 minutes, and in the control group - 90270 minutes, on average 180.9±35.7 minutes.

Patients who underwent BAC had a skin incision length of 2.03.0 cm, averaging 3.0±0.9 cm, while the control group had a skin incision length of 4.0-6.0 cm, averaging4.3±2.6 cm. We did not note any intraoperative complications in any patient of both groups.

During the study period, a total of 60 interintestinal anastomoses were performed in newborns (24 (40%) in the main group and 36 (60%) in the control group): of them end-to-end anastomosis was 50 (83.3%), side-to-side anastomosis 1 (1.7%) and end-to-side anastomosis 9 (15%). Two-row continuous suture with absorbable suture material *VICRYL (VICRYL) 5/0-6/0* was considered to be the technique of choice for interintestinal access in newborns in both groups.

When the obstruction was localised at the level of the jejunum and ileum, the indications for a particular type of anastomosis were determined depending on the nature of the malformation, its complications, and the difference in the diameters of the driving and diverting segments. The most physiological is the end-to-end interintestinal anastomosis, which was used in 50 (44.2%) cases of jejunal and ileum atresia.

The main indication for end-to-side anastomosis was a large difference in the ratio between the driving and the withdrawing end of the small intestine.

The absolute indications for the removal of double-barrel stoma were cases of ileum atresia on the background of perforation and spilled peritonitis. In addition, enterostomies were removed in cases of small intestinal atresia, as intrauterine inflammation of the intestinal wall limits the interintestinal junction.

The volume of resection depended on the level of atresia and the severity of secondary changes in the atresised segment. According to literature data based on morphological studies, the degree and extent of the lesion of the suprastenotic dilated zone depends on the level of malformation localisation: the lower the atresia is located, the more pronounced are the destructive changes. This fact is explained by the impossibility of emptying the dilated parts during vomiting or gastric probing. Therefore, in atresia at the level of jejunum the resection of the driving loop was usually performed within 7-10 cm, the diverting one - 5-7 cm, in atresia at the level of ileum the driving segment was resected within 10-20 cm, the diverting one - 5-7 cm. The volume of resection in necrotic lesions of the intestine was determined by the extent of the changed areas.

In the main group, postoperative bowel paresis was noted 24-48 hours, while in the control group - 4-5 days. In patients with weak peristalsis in the early postoperative period from 3 days onwards, intestinal function was stimulated by injecting 5 ml of saline solution through a naso- or orogastroduodenal tube, 0.05-0.1 ml of 0.05% proserine solution was injected intramuscularly, and electrophoresis with lidase was applied through the anterior abdominal wall.

In 4-5 hours after surgery, the decompression probe was extended to restore duodenal motility. At first, distilled water or ORSA solution was infused, then mixtures, in the ratio of 1:4 at first, later 1:2, then 3:4 to the full volume.

In the absence of mother's milk, special formula for newborns (NAN, Nutrilak, HIPP, Malyutka, etc.) and premature infants (Alfare, PreNAN, Pregestemilk) were used. Weight gain in dynamics was considered as a criterion for normalisation of the patient's general condition.

The period of children's stay in OARIT was significantly reduced (to 7-10 days), whereas after laparotomy this indicator was 17-24 days. The duration of hospital stay after video-assisted operations was 7-10 days, on average 7.4±2.2 days, and after open operations - 17-24 days, on average 17.3±1.8 days.

In the postoperative period, early activation of patients was observed within 3-4 days after surgery using video-assisted technique. Comparison of postoperative complications by groups is presented in Figure 4.11.

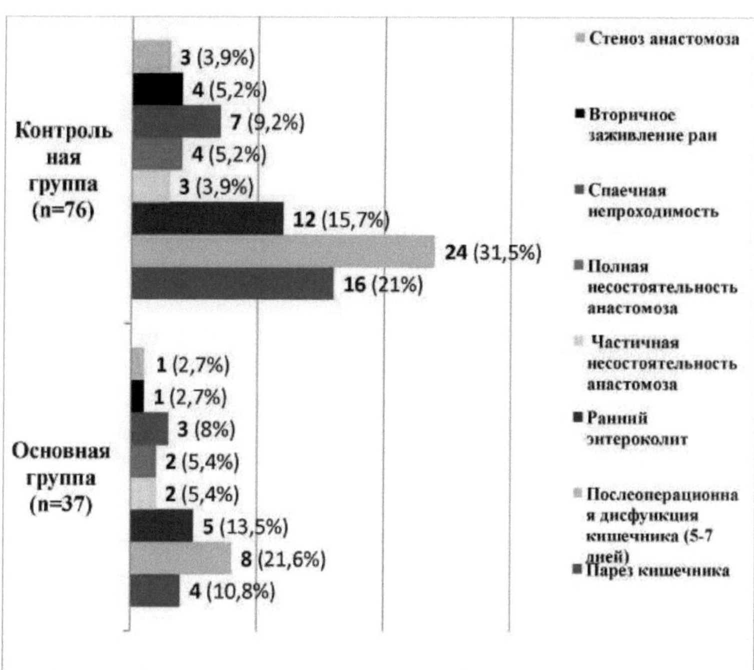

Fig.4.11. Comparative characteristics of early postoperative complications by groups

Our study showed that gross complications in neonates with EIA were: 22.1% in the main group 8(7.1%), in the control group - 17(15%). The mortality rate among children with EIA was23%: 5(4.4%) in the main group and 21(18.6%) in the control group.

The presence of multiple malformations and somatic conditions in the patients most accurately affected the outcome of treatment and this is summarised in Figure 4.12.

ЛЕТАЛЬНЫЙ ИСХОД (n=26) 23%
Доношенный 9 (34,6%)
Недоношенный 17 (65,4%)
Основная группа 5 (19,2%)
Контрольная группа 21 (80,8%)
Дон. 1 (3,8%)
Недон. 4 (15,4%)
Дон. 8 (30,8%)
Недон. 13 (50%)

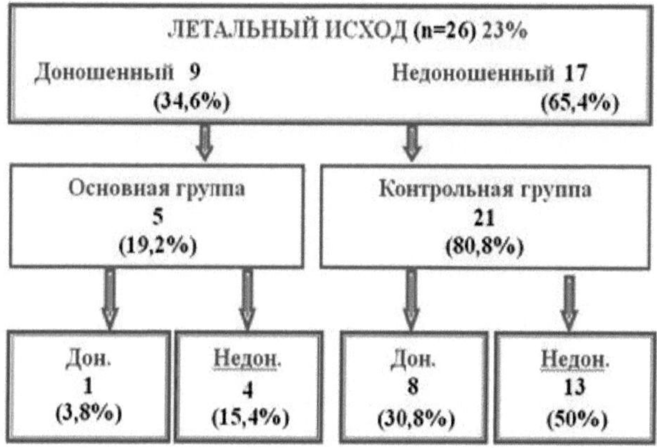

Fig.4.12.Results of lethal outcome in neonates with EIA

Analysis of the results suggests that surgical aggression in VAS is significantly lower than traditional methods.

We also studied the *long-term results of treatment of* patients with EIA (on average 2 years after surgery). Out of 37 operated (EIA) children, we were able to evaluate the long-term results in 29 (78.4%) cases, in four cases it was not possible due to the patients' death (the other four did not agree due to family circumstances). The cause of this outcome, according to our data, was malabsorption syndrome. We used a questionnaire survey with 29 parents to evaluate the long-term results. We developed a questionnaire form consisting of a list of questions with answer options (Table 4.3.).

Table 4.3. Form of questionnaires of distant results in patients.

Indicators	Answer options	Score	Results (n=29)
Current health status of the child time	completely healthy	1	
	satisfactory	2	
	unsatisfactory	3	
	yes	1	
	diet	2	
Can eat any kind of food	mixture	3	
	no	1	
Stools (number of times per day)	1 time	2	
	more than 2-3 times	3	
Vomiting	No	1	
	once a day	2	
	1-2 times a month	3	
Spontaneous abdominal pain	no	1	
	occasionally	2	
	frequently	3	
Weight and height gain	age-appropriate	1	
	sometimes yes, sometimes no.	2	
	underweight	3	
Surgical wound	With primary healing	1	
	With secondary healing	2	
	Fistula formation	3	

If the child scored 7-10, the condition was assessed as satisfactory, from 11-17 score - moderate severity, above 17 - severe condition, in this case the child should be hospitalised.Out of 29 patients 22(76%) scored from 7-10, 5(17.2%) scored from 1117 and 2(6.8%) above 17 score.

Here is an example. *Patient M.N.(f.m.) born 27.12.2018, I/B No. 1235 was admitted to the Republican Training and Methodological Centre for Neonatal Surgery at the*

RTC from the neonatal department on 27.12.2018. Antenatally diagnosed with GI tract abnormalities. GI tract, complaints of vomiting with bile, lack of stool and abdominal bloating.

According to the medical ***history****, the newborn started vomiting bile from birth. After birth, the child was examined by a neonatal surgeon at the RRC and diagnosed with "GI tract malformation. GI TRACT. ICH". He was referred for surgical treatment at the RRCNH at the RRC in the OARIT.*

Anamnesisvitae: *according to mother's words, the child of III pregnancy III child; male. Pregnancy was accompanied by toxicosis, acute respiratory infections and anaemia. Delivery at 34 weeks, physiological; birth weight - 2700 g, received prophylactic vaccinations; mother and father are related.*

On examination, the general condition of the patient in the main disease is very severe. Skin and visible mucous membranes are clean, pale pink in colour. Subcutaneous fatty fibre is moderately developed. Body temperature is 36.9 C. Physiological reflexes are evoked. There are no deformities in the musculoskeletal system. Breathing is independent, through the nose. No deformities are found in the thorax. Hard breathing is heard auscultatively in the lungs. The apex of the cardiac tone is located 1.0 lateral to the Linea media clavicularis sinistra. Cardiac tones are rhythmic. Not fed. Abdomen is distended, symmetrically involved in the act of breathing; painless, soft on palpation. The liver and spleen are not enlarged. Auscultatory intestinal peristalsis is heard weakly. Stool does not pass. Urination is independent.

Statuslocalis: an *orogastric tube was inserted, which passed into the stomach without obstruction. The probe expelled 110.0 ml of pathological fluid with bile (Fig.3.13).Abdominal bloating slightly decreased, painless, soft on palpation; auscultatory intestinal peristalsis is heard weakly; stool did not pass, stimulation reveals a "mucous plug" (Fig.4.13).*

*Laboratory investigations were carried out. In the general blood count haemoglobin up to 190 g/l, erythrocytes 7.4 g/l*10. Blood biochemistry without pathological phenomena. Blood coagulogram is normal.*

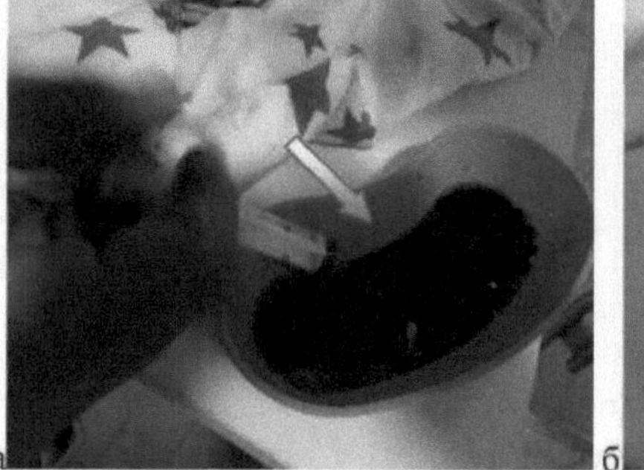

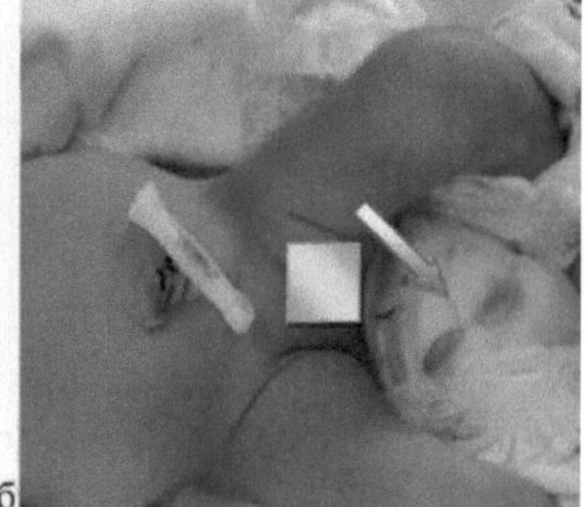

Fig.4.13. Clinical signs of VTCN in a newborn. Patient M.N. (f.m) I/B.1235. a) contents with bile comes out through the orogastric tube; b) "mucous plug"

comes out during stimulation of the anus

Instrumental investigations. *NSG: dilatation of external liquor passages on the background of hypoxia. EchoCG: open oval window 3.5 mm, additional chorda in LV; heart chambers were not dilated, no signs of inflammation. Ultrasound of internal organs: loop of intestine dilated to 6.0 cm, other abdominal organs without echopathology.*

Review radiography of the abdominal cavity: incomplete pneumatisation of the abdominal cavity (Fig.4.14.a.). Contrast irrigography: in the direct projection at full filling of the large intestine the symptom of "small intestine" is determined (Fig. 4.14.6.).

An anaesthesiologist and intensive care specialist examined the patient and recommended emergency surgical treatment. No contraindications to video-assisted surgery were identified in the patient after laboratory, clinical and paraclinical investigations.

A clinical diagnosis has *been established. Primary: congenital malformation of the GI tract. ICH. in the initial part of the small intestine. Associated: aspiration bronchopneumonia. Background: 34 weeks premature. The patient was prepared for video-assisted operation on the small intestine as an emergency.*

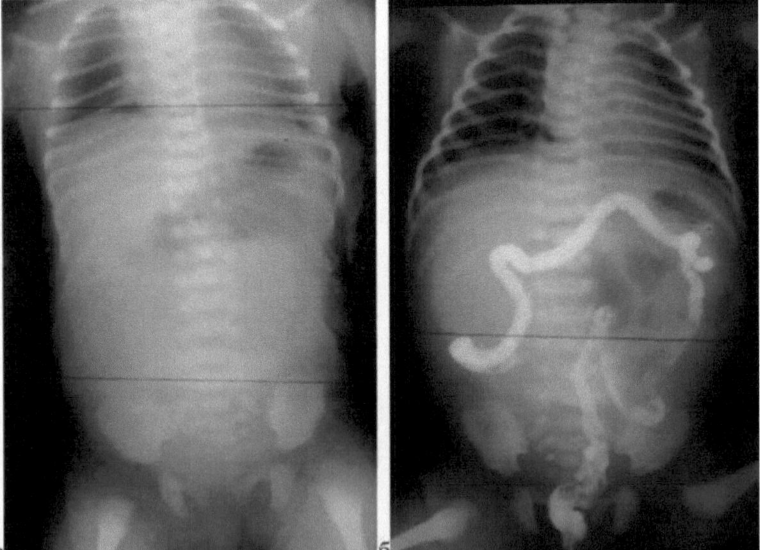

Fig.4.14. Radiographic examination of the abdominal cavity in direct projection. Patient M.N. (f.m) I/B.1235.a) Review radiography of the abdominal cavity; decreased pneumatisation, horizontal level, "mute abdomen" in the lower abdominal cavity. b) Irrigogram (Triombrast 76%-10.0 + Sodium chlorine 0.9% - 10.0 ml)- the symptom of "small intestine" is positive.

Course of the operation. *Under intubation anaesthesia in the supine position after treatment of the operative field in the infraumbilical region, the first trocar with a diameter of 2 mm was placed, CO2 insufflation was performed and pneumoperitoneum was created. Further, a trocar (3.0 mm) to the right of the umbilicus was placed with a HOPKINSII5 mm rod under the control of the optics. Revision of the abdominal cavity revealed adhesions. The adhesions were disconnected with a bipolar coagulator. An atresised part of the small intestine was found 15 cm from the proximal part of the ligament of Tracey's ligament, the distal end in the form of a "cord". The correspondence between the driving and withdrawing ends is 5:1. A mesenteric defect is identified.*

A 2.5 cm minilararatomic incision was made at the trocar site on the right side and the atresised part of the jejunum was removed. The patency of the diverting end of the intestine was checked. On revision, 4 atresised parts were identified in the area of jejunal atresia every 5-7cm. We resected from the initial atresised part of the jejunum to the fourth atresised area, approximately 25cm of jejunum was resected. A nasogastric tube (#6) was passed for intestinal intubation. Next, the driving end of the jejunum was narrowed to match the diameter of the bowel with the diverting end of the bowel. An inter-intestinal anastomosis was applied and sutured with single-row sutures (PDS #5.0). The tightness was checked. The mesenteric defect was sutured with Vicryl #5.0. Then the intestinal loops were carefully immersed into the abdominal cavity. The abdominal cavity was drained through the laparotome opening. Haemostasis in the course of the operation. Layer sutures on the wound. Iodine. Alcohol. Aseptic dressing. The macropreparation was sent for histological examination.

Histological examination of the macro preparation: *Resected diverting part of the jejunum 25.0 cm long, 4.0 - atresized part, driving part of the jejunum (3 cm), part funnel-shaped dilated (Fig. 4.15).*

Postoperative course *was smooth. He received antibacterial therapy (cefepime, vancomycin), haemostatic drugs (Vitamin K), complete parenteral nutrition up to 3 days. Intestinal stimulation (metoclopramide 0.1 ml/kg), enteral feeding via intestinal tube were started on the 3rd day. On the 5th day microclysemia with hypertonic solution was added to intestinal stimulation.*

On the 6th day there was an independent stool, after which feeding through an orogastric tube was added. The interstinal tube (intubator) was released every other day by 1.0-1.5 cm. According to the patient's condition, in case of satisfactory defecation the interstinal tube was removed. Before removal of the interstinal probe, the patient underwent GI passage, the contrast agent (triombrast 76%) passed without obstruction through the anastomosis zone at 120 minutes after the passage.

A partial 2:1 correspondence between the driving and withdrawing ends of the intestine was preserved. On the 14th day the child was discharged home in satisfactory condition. At discharge, the surgical wound was primary healed, and the sutures were removed. Electrophoresis of the anterior abdominal wall with alternation of proserin and lidaza for 10 days on the 15th-20th day after the operation was recommended. Obligatory follow-up at the place of residence with a neonatologist (gastroenterologist).

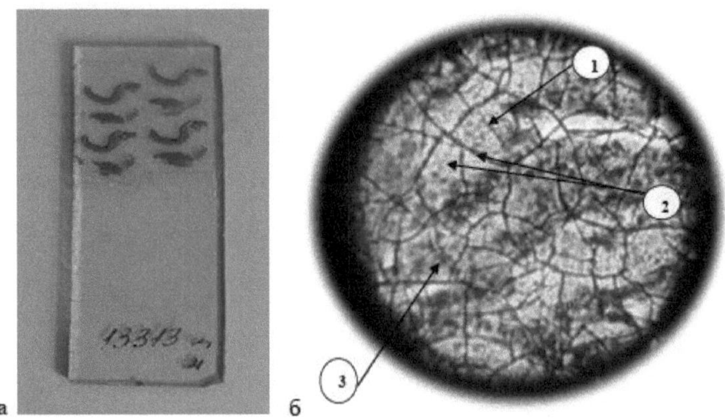

Fig.4.15. Patient M.N., (f.m.) I/B No. 1235: a) macroprepath; b) microscopy photo of the patient's jejunum. Reduced lumen diameter and submucosal fibrosis (1 arrow). The jejunal muscles show hypertrophy of annular muscles (2 arrow) without ganglionic plexus.

Atrophy of crypts of jejunum, villi of jejunum (3 arrow).

The radiograph shows that the contrast agent is gradually evacuated into the colon without delay(Fig.4.16).

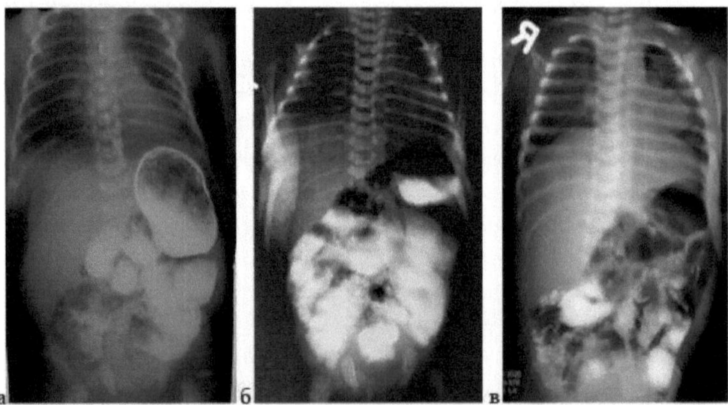

Fig. 4.16. Patient M.N. (f.m.) I/B No. 1235. After video-assisted small bowel surgery. The child was examined with GI tract passage 1 month after discharge: a) at 60 minutes; b) 120 minutes; c) 180 minutes.

The use of video-assisted laparoscopy can achieve excellent cosmetic results with minimal surgical procedures injuries (Figure 4.17).

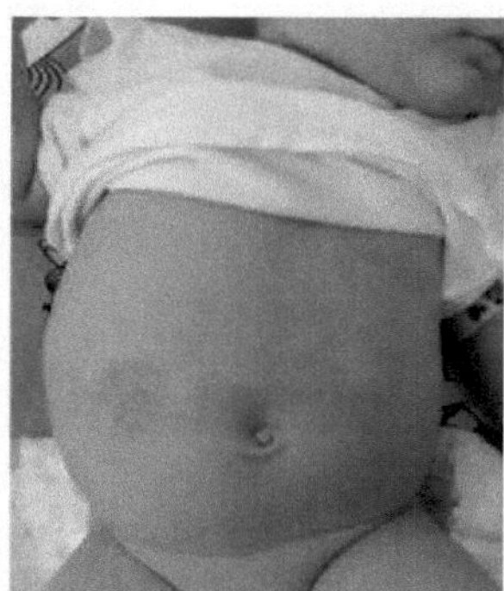

Fig.4.17. Patient M.N. (f.m.) I/B #1235 with VTCN 1 month after video-assisted small bowel surgery: anterior abdominal wall.

The long-term follow-up of our patients demonstrated the reliability of laparoscopic access, which was confirmed by the favourable course of the postoperative period and the absence of disease recurrence regardless of the type of congenital anomaly.

Indications and contraindications for video-assisted laparascopy in neonates.

Indications for video-assisted laparascopy.

Today, diagnostic laparoscopy is in the stage of active development. This method of diagnosis makes it possible to choose the correct treatment tactics, to perform radical surgical intervention without laparotomy.

Contraindications to video-assisted laparascopy.

Diagnostic laparoscopy is a minimally invasive surgical procedure. Therefore, contraindications to this procedure should be taken seriously. There are absolute and relative contraindications. Video-assisted laparoscopy is strictly forbidden in case of haemorrhagic shock caused by severe blood loss.

Contraindications to video-assisted surgery are intrauterine and postnatal generalised intrauterine peritonitis, prematurity (III-IV degree), low gestational age and excessive intestinal bloating. In our study we met 8(7%) extremely premature (6 had grade III and 2 had grade IV prematurity) babies. We refused to operate them by video-assisted surgery because most of the complications are related to dysfunction of immature systems and organs. For example, underdevelopment of the respiratory centre in the brainstem leads to apnoea attacks, rapid development of necrotizing enterocolitis with painful bloating of the abdomen.

Static processing of the study results

Benefits of video-assisted surgery:

- good cosmetic effect
- relative paucity
- low traumatisation
- the magnification the video camera gives.

Disadvantages of video-assisted surgery:

- technological complexity
- the need for skills in the surgeon
- small abdominal volume in neonates and therefore the use of adapted instruments
- creation of prolonged pneumoperitoneum, which negatively affects lung excursion;
- high cost

Advantages of minilaparotomy:

- excellent cosmetic results;
- simplicity of technological execution;
- there is no need for prolonged pneumoperitoneum.

When surgical interventions were performed using the VAM technique, newborns were placed in the intensive care unit for 10-15 days, enteral feeding was started from the 5th day, and the children were given adequate infusion and antibacterial therapy. After normalisation and strengthening of the condition, the children were transferred to the surgical department, from where they were discharged home in satisfactory condition on the 25-28th day.

Summary of the chapter

The analysis of surgical correction of EIA in newborns allows us to conclude that the introduction of a new method of surgical correction contributes to the reduction of early postoperative complications and mortality.

Timely diagnosis, adequate preoperative preparation and postoperative management of neonates with jejunoileal atresia, taking into account all factors that can aggravate the course of the disease and the postoperative period, can not only improve the course of the postoperative period, but also reduce mortality.

Thus, the choice of the method of surgical root canalisation depends mainly on the experience of the paediatric surgeon, clinical features and concomitant pathologies. The prognosis depends to a greater extent on the type of atresia according to the histopathological picture of the affected intestine.

The study confirms that in terms of preventing early postoperative complications such as anastomosis failure and peritonitis, the recommended surgical method is more effective than traditional surgical techniques.

The use of modern treatment techniques, development of algorithms for diagnosis and treatment of small bowel atresia allowed to reduce the mortality rate of newborns with EIA from 42% to 26%.

In case of large ratios between the driving and diverting parts of the small intestine, primary anastomosis should be sought, including narrowing of the driving segment. According to the technique of interintestinal anastomosis in newborns, the method of choice is the double-row continuous suture with synthetic absorbable suture *material VICRYL (VICRYL) 5/0-6/0*, which has proven its advantage in practice, both in terms of simplicity and reliability.

CONCLUSION

Analysis of literature data on modern aspects of embryogenesis, epidemiology and diagnosis of EIA shows that the definition of criteria for antenatal diagnosis of fetal SCCI is extremely important. Early ante- and postnatal diagnosis, adequate assessment of the severity of the condition of children with VTCN has not only theoretical but also practical importance and requires the development of new methodological positions. The high incidence of postoperative complications makes it urgent to improve the methods of surgical correction of this malformation.

An integrated approach to pre- and postnatal diagnosis and treatment of neonatal ileal atresia will help to give a correct assessment of the clinical picture of the disease and predict the course of the intra- and postoperative period, possible complications and improve the results of correction of this malformation.

The present scientific study is the result of many years of work of the Republican Training and Methodological Centre for Neonatal Surgery under the ROC, the clinical base of the Department of Hospital Paediatric Surgery of the Tashkent Children's Medical Institute in the field of neonatal EIA surgery. Many surgical interventions performed within the framework of the study were performed for the first time in the Republic of Uzbekistan. The accumulated experience made it possible to create the largest database of patients who underwent surgical correction of EIA during the newborn period.

The aim of the study is to improve the results of surgical treatment of congenital small intestinal atresia in newborns by selecting the most optimal diagnostic and surgical methods.

In accordance with the objective, the following tasks have been defined:

To determine the most characteristic echographic signs and risk factors for the development of congenital small intestinal obstruction in the foetus, taking into account the results of antenatal diagnosis;

To develop obstetric tactics with clear indications and contraindications for preservation or termination of pregnancy in different types of congenital small intestinal obstruction in the foetus, taking into account associated malformations;

Analyse diagnostic errors at the level of maternity wards and develop a diagnostic algorithm for congenital small intestinal obstruction in newborns;

to study the clinical picture and determine the proportion of this anomaly in the structure of other malformations;

To develop indications and contraindications for video-assisted operations in congenital small intestinal obstruction in newborns, taking into account concomitant malformations and somatic background;

To determine the most effective method of surgical correction by comparative analysis of the immediate and long-term results of conventional and video-assisted operations for congenital small intestinal obstruction in newborns.

The study analysed the results of diagnosis and surgical correction of 113 neonates with EIA in ROC in 2014 - 2021.

The analysis was performed in all (n=113) newborns admitted with a diagnosis of VTCN in the period from 2014 to 2021, assessing the course of pregnancy and somatic status of the mothers, as well as the results of tests. We also analysed the data obtained from the anamnesis of the newborn, taking into account clinical and anamnestic indicators, transport conditions and the results of diagnostic tests performed both in the maternity hospital and in a specialised hospital.

The analysis showed that newborns were hospitalised in the first 24 hours of life in 73.5%, 1-3 days in 19.5%, and later in 7% of cases, respectively, indicating a low level of early diagnosis of VTCN in maternity hospitals.

The most significant frequent risk factors were ARVI in early pregnancy in 92%, medication in 76%, threat of miscarriage in 68%; anaemia in 54%, environmental factors in 39%, and TOXN infection in 18.5%, respectively.

Adequate diagnosis both antenatally and postnatally, assessment of the patient's condition, proper intensive care at the maternity hospital and compliance with all transport rules play a major role in the favourable outcome of patients with VTCN.

The results of the study showed that in43 (38%) cases the rules of interhospital transport were violated: the newborns were not given the necessary therapeutic measures, which led to destabilisation of the newborns' condition.

The analysis showed that only adequate preparation in maternity hospitals with all necessary diagnostic measures and transport were observed in53(47%) cases. In 18(16%) cases, the neonates were not given all the necessary measures during transport leading to destabilisation of the condition. All the above resulted in patients admitted in hypothermia (<36.0°C) in 21(18.6%); hyperthermia (>37.5°C) in 8(7%) cases respectively. Newborns were admitted in severe condition in 11.5% of cases and in extremely severe condition in 2.6%.

Taking into account the above, we proposed an algorithm for the management of neonates with VTCN both antenatally and postnatally. For convenience, we divided the patients into two groups.

The control group included37 children with EIA who were treated in 2017-2021 and underwent video-assisted surgery with minilaparatomic incision. We analysed the results of diagnosis and treatment of newborns in the main group, which allowed us to change the approaches to diagnosis and treatment of patients with EIA.

In the control group, primary small intestine anastomosis was performed in 47 (60%) newborns, and enterostomy was removed in 34 (43.5%). The anastomosis was performed in the traditional way, i.e. single and double row knotted sutures. In the main group, primary small intestine anastomosis was performed in 27(77%) children, and enterostomy was removed in 8(23%) newborns.

The mortality in the postoperative period among the control group patients was 27%. Septic and haemorrhagic causes against the background of postoperative complications (anastomosis failure, peritonitis) can be distinguished among the reasons for this. Early postoperative complications developed in 18 (23.6%) out of 76 patients. The largest percentage of them was postoperative intestinal dysfunction

24(31.5%), secondary wound healing - 24(31.5%),
Small intestine anastomosis failure - 19(25%).

In the main group, postoperative complications developed in 5 (14.2%) cases. Lethality was due to septic and haemorrhagic causes. The most frequent complication was postoperative intestinal dysfunction - 8(21.6%), secondary wound healing - 1(2.7%), small intestine anastomosis failure - 6(16.2%).

Thus, the analysis of mortality in the postoperative period in both groups showed that in the main group mortality was 5(13.5%), cases against 21(27%) in the control group.

conclusions

- The main echographic signs of fetal small intestinal atresia in the antenatal period are: polyuria (100%), dilatation of the small intestinal loops by more than 15 mm in the second trimester of pregnancy (100%), which is manifested by the presence of multiple "bubbles" in the abdominal cavity of the foetus. Of these, multihydroids is the most significant and easily identifiable antenatal sign, requiring mandatory postnatal examination of the newborn for bowel anomaly. The reliability of antenatal ultrasound diagnosis of fetal small bowel atresia is 59%.
- In antenatal diagnosis of fetal intestinal malformations, obstetric tactics should be decided in conjunction with neonatal surgeons and other relevant specialists (cardiac surgeon, neurosurgeon, etc.). Obstetric tactics in foetal intestinal peritonitis depends on the presence of complications in the form of intrauterine peritonitis, as well as combined and multiple malformations.
- Antenatal diagnosis of fetal intestinal malformations requires an active search for combined and other anomalies. The detection of uncorrectable and gross multiple anomalies in a foetus with SCCN is an indication for termination of pregnancy. Small intestinal atresia is often combined with malformations of the MBC (30.4%) and cardiovascular system (27%).
- Risk factors for fetal small intestinal atresia in 92 per cent of cases

was associated with acute respiratory pathology, 68% with early pregnancy termination threat, 18.5% with TORCH infection, 54% with anaemia, 76% with teratogenic effects of medications and 39% with adverse environmental factors. The vast majority of pregnant women (38%) have 3 or more of the above risk factors.

- The most common diagnostic and tactical errors are made by

in maternity institutions and at the stages of routing of newborns with intestinal atresia. In 55.8% of cases, these patients are admitted to a specialised surgical department in a serious condition due to late diagnosis. Only 34.5% of children are diagnosed on the first day of life, while 26.5% of patients are diagnosed on the second day or later. At the same time, aspiration pneumonia was verified in 100% of cases.

- The main early clinical manifestations of UTI in newborns are vomiting with intestinal contents (100%), discharge of uncoloured mucous plugs (100%) and abdominal bloating (76%). The share of this anomaly in the structure of other malformations is 4% and 41.6% among NSCLC.
- Video-assisted surgery is the method of choice for surgical correction of VTCN in newborns, which significantly reduces postoperative complications. Contraindications to video-assisted surgery are intrauterine meconium and postnatal spilled peritonitis, low gestational age (28 weeks and below) and profound prematurity, as well as excessive abdominal bloating.
- The advantages of video-assisted surgery for neonatal VTCN are minimal contact of internal organs with the external environment, early extubation (on the 2nd day), 2-fold reduction of hospital stay, reduction of pain syndrome and minimal postoperative

complications in the form of suppuration, hernia and adhesions. Video-assisted operations allowed to reduce mortality from 27% in the comparison group to 13.5% in the main group, i.e. 2 times.

PRACTICAL RECOMMENDATIONS

1. Prenatal ultrasound diagnostics in dynamics, taking into account the identified risk factors for the formation of foetal EIA, makes it possible to conduct a targeted search for this malformation at an earlier gestational age and thereby improve prenatal diagnosis of EIA;
2. Application of the algorithms of ante- and postnatal diagnostics and tactics of management of newborns with EIA developed in the clinic allows to detect this defect in the first hours of the child's life, helps to reduce complications associated with late detection, as well as to choose the optimal therapeutic tactics and improve the results of surgical treatment.
3. The use of video-assisted surgery allows to significantly reduce postoperative complications, achieve a good result with minimal surgical trauma and a favourable course of the postoperative period of patients with jejunoileal atresia.

REFERENCE LIST

1. Akselrov M.A. Artificial intestinal fistulas in abdominal surgery in children: autoref. diss. Dr. of medical sciences: 14.01.19 /Akselrov Mikhail Aleksandrovich. - M., 2012. - 44 c.

2. Akselrov M.A. Low intestinal obstruction. Approach to treatment/ M.A. Axelrov, V.V. Ivanov, S.N. Suprunets // Bulletin of Russian State Medical University. - 2010.- №3. - C. 8.

3. Amidkhonova S.A. Criteria for the choice of the method of anastomosis creation in newborns with small intestinal obstruction: autorref. Cand. Sciences: spets. 14.01.19/ Amidkhonova Suraye Azimkhonovna. - Ufa, 2015. - 214 c.

4. Aprosimov M.N. Laparotomy in surgery of congenital intestinal obstruction / M.N.Aprosimov // Bulletin of Russian State Medical University. - 2010. - № 3. - C. 5859.

5. Baibarina, E.H.. Improvement of early surgical care for children with congenital malformations / E.H. Baibarina, D.N. Degtyarev, Yu. Baibarina, D.N. Degtyarev, Y.I. Kucherov // Russian Herald of Perinatology and Paediatrics. - 2011. - №2. - C. 12-19.

6. Baigulov, M.S. Justification and development of methods for assessing the organisation of surgical care for children with congenital malformations of the gastrointestinal tract: autoref. diss. ... Dr. of medical sciences / Baigulov Mamadiyar Shayzadaevich. - Astana, 2011. - 20 c.

7. Baigulov M.Sh. Justification and development of methods for assessing the organisation of surgical care for children with congenital malformations of the GI tract// Dissertation work. National Scientific Centre of Maternity and Childhood Astana. 2011. - 3 pp. [Electronic resource] URL: httpshttps://pandia.ru/text/79/501/47976-3.phppandia.ru/text/79/501/47976-3.php (date of reference: 15.05.2021).

8. Criteria for choosing the method of anastomosis in newborns with small intestinal obstruction / V.G. Bairov, S.A. Amidkhanova, N.A.
Shchegoleva and [et al.]// Paediatric Surgery. - 2015. - T. 19. - № 1. - C. 1520.

9. Batchenko N.Y. Surgical treatment of newborns with small intestine atresia / N.Y. Batchenko, O.G. Mokrushina, A.A. Gogichaeva // Russian journal of paediatric surgery, anaesthesiology and resuscitation.
- 2020. - T. 10. - № 4. - C. 473-486. https://doi.org/10.17816/ psaic639.

10. Botviniev, O.K.. Comparative characteristics of phenogenotypic features in newborns with atresia of the duodenum and other parts of the small intestine / O.K. Botviniev, A.V. Eremeeva // Russian Journal of Gastroenterology, Hepatology, Coloproctology. Botviniev, A.V. Eremeeva // Russian Journal of Gastroenterology, Hepatology, Coloproctology. - 2012. - T. 22, № 3. - C. 20-25.

11. Congenital intestinal obstruction. Choice of surgical tactics and intestinal suture technique / V.A. Savvina, A.R. Varfolomeev, M.E. Okhlopkov, V.N. Nikolaev // Far Eastern Medical Journal. -2012.-№4.-C. 3740.

12. Congenital small intestinal obstruction [Electronic resource] // SurgeryZone.

Medical site . - Access mode:
http ://surgeryzone. net/detskaya-xirurgiya/vrozhdennaya-neproxodimost-tonkoj - kishki.html. - Downloaded from the screen.
13. T-shaped intestinal anastomosis in neonatal surgery / V.N. Grona, G.A. Sopov, C.B. Vesely [et al. Vesely [et al] // Bulletin of Russian State Medical University. - 2010. -№ 3. - C. 15.
14. To the issue of prevention of recurrence of adhesive intestinal obstruction in children / A.E. Erekeshov, Y.M. Olkhovik, E.A. Musin [et al.] // Vestnik of Emergency and Restorative Medicine. - 2008. - T. 9. - № 3. -C. 432433.
15. Features of surgical correction of congenital small intestinal obstruction: a clinical and experimental study / A. S. Zheleznov, N. S. Ermolaeva, L. A. Separate, [et al.]// Modern Problems of Science and Education ;
URL: https://science-education.ru/ru/article/view?id=29565.
16. Recovery of a newborn with multiple segmental necrosis of the intestine / I.P. Zhurilo, V.P. Perunsky, A.B. Shcherbinin, A.A. Muzalev // Clinical anatomy and operative surgery. Shcherbinin, A.A. Muzalev // Clinical anatomy and operative surgery. - 2007. - T. 6. - № 3. - C. 29-33.
17. Method of laparoscopic decompression of the small intestine in intestinal obstruction and peritonitis in children / A.N. Izosimov, A.A. Gumerov, V.V. Plechev [et al. Plechev [et al] // Medical Bulletin of Bashkortostan. -2012.-T. 7. - №2.- C. 97-99.
18. Neonatal surgery [Text] / [Averyanova Y. V. et al.] ; ed. by Y. F. Isakov, N. N. Volodin, A. V. Geraskin. - Moscow: Dynasty, 2011. - 687 c. : ill.; 24 cm.
19. Congenital malformations of the gastrointestinal tract as a joint problem of paediatric surgeons and paediatricians / I.Yu. Karpova, V.V. Parshikov, A.C. Zheleznov [et al] // Medical Almanac. - 2010. -№4.- C. 208-210.
20. Katko V.A. Gastrointestinal tract obstruction in children / V.A. Katko. - Minsk, 2010. - 153 c.
21. Katsupeev, V.B. Single-row suture in abdominal anastomoses in children over a month old / V.B. Katsupeev // Children's Surgery. - 2012. - № 5. - C. 22-25.
22. The role of entero-colostomy in the pathology of the gastrointestinal tract in infants / A.A. Kashitsyna [et al] // Bulletin of Surgery. I.I.Grekov.- 2010 № 4.-P. 123.
23. Kenzhebaeva K.A.Structure of gastrointestinal tract atresia in newborns and their survival rate in this pathology / K.A. Kenzhebaeva, I.V. Kumeiko, M.A. Borisevich, A.M. Izenov [et al.]// (Kazakhstan) Medicine and Ecology. - 2019. - №1. - C. 59-65.
24. Atresia of the digestive tract: a guide for doctors / ed. by Y. A. Kozlov, A. Y. Razumovsky, V. A. Novozhilov [et al]. - Moscow: GEOTAR-Media, 2021. - 416 p.: ill.
25. Modern strategies of surgical treatment of small intestine atresia / Yu.A. Kozlov, V.A. Novozhilov, A.B. Podkamenev [et al. Podkamenev [et al] // Russian journal of paediatric surgery, anaesthesiology and resuscitation. - 2010. - № 1. -c. 42-48.
26. Laparoscopic anastomosis in small intestine atresia / Yu. A. Kozlov, A.A.

Rasputin, K.A. Kovalkov // Paediatric Surgery. - 2019. - T. 23. - № 6. - C. 335-338. - URL:https://doi.org/10.https://doi.org/10.18821/1560-9510-2019-23-6-335- 338
27. Laparoscopic treatment for small intestine atresia / Yu.A. Kozlov, A.A. Rasputin, K.A. Kovalkov [et al] // Endoscopic Surgery. *-2020.* -T. 26. - №3.- C. 47-51.
28. Kulakov V.I. Emergency surgical correction of congenital malformations in newborns / V.I. Kulakov // Obstetrics and Gynaecology. - 2009. - № 3. - C. 47-50.
29. Kucherov Yu.I., Dorofeeva E.I. Experience of treatment of patients with congenital intestinal obstruction in the perinatal centre / Yu.I. Kucherov, E.I. Dorofeeva // Children's Surgery. - 2009. - № 5. - C. 11-16.
30. Losev, A.A. Experience of treatment of newborns with artificial intestinal fistulas / A.A. Losev[et al] // Neonatology, Surgery, Perinatal Medicine. - 2013. - T. 7. - № 5. - C. 47-50.
31. Results of surgical treatment of children with congenital intestinal obstruction / N.M.Lysyakov,S.A.MarkosyashchN.A.Okunev [et al.] // Practical Medicine. - 2008. - № 6. - C. 72.
32. Makarova MA, Lyaturinskaya OV Treatment of newborns with small intestinal atresia / MA Makarova MA, OV Lyaturinskaya // Surgery of Childhood. - 2013. - № 2. - C. 6-10.
33. Mamleyev, I.A.; Alibaev, A.K. New approaches to the diagnosis and treatment of early adhesion obstruction in children / I.A. Mamleyev, A.K. Alibaev // Reproductive health of children and adolescents. - 2007. - № 4. - C. 86-91.
34. Markosyan S.A., Okunev N.A. Results of surgical treatment of children with congenital intestinal obstruction / S.A. Markosyan, N.A. Okunev // Bulletin of Russian State Medical University. - 2010. - № 3. - C. 30
35. Mashinets N.V. Demidov V.N., Kucherov Yu.I. Opportunities of echography in prenatal diagnosis of small and large intestine atresia / N.V. Mashinets, V.N. Demidov, Yu.I. Kucherov // Prenatal Diagnostics. - 2010. -T. 9. - № 1. - C. 20-24
36. Medvedev, M. V. Prenatal echography: differential diagnosis and prognosis / M. V. Medvedev. - 3rd ed., supplement, revision. - Moscow: Real Time, 2012. - 448 p.: ill., tab., coloured ill.; 29 cm.; ISBN 978-5-903025-46-6 (in Russian).
37. Congenital atresia of the gastrointestinal tract in newborns / M.A. Borisevich, I.D. Kumeiko, A.M. Izenov // International Journal of Applied and Fundamental Research. - 2019. - № 6. - C. 78-84. - URL: httpshttps://applied-research.ru/ru/article/view7idM2771applied-research.ru/ru/article/view7idM2771 (date of reference: 26.04.2023).
38. Mironov, P.I. Relationship of systemic inflammatory response with the nature of nutritional support during surgery in children with early adhesion obstruction / P.I. Mironov, V.U. Sataev // Russian journal of paediatric surgery, anaesthesiology and resuscitation. - 2014. - T. 4, №2.-C. 58-62.
39. Comparative analysis of surgical treatment of duodenal obstruction in newborns / O.G. Mokrushina, A.B. Geraskin, N.V. Golodenko [et al. Geraskin, N.V. Golodenko [et al] // Russian journal of paediatric surgery, anaesthesiology and resuscitation. -

2010. - № 1. - C. 49-53.
40. The role of laparoscopy in the diagnosis of acquired bowel disease Obstruction in newborns and infants / O.G. Mokrushina, N.V. Golodenko, M.V. Levitskaya [et al.] // Medical Bulletin of the North Caucasus. - 2009. - T. 13, № 1. - C. 42Ь.
41. Comparative characteristics of methods of surgical treatment of meconium peritonitis in newborns / V.I. Morozov, A.A.
Podshivalin, M.A. Zykova [et al] // Practical Medicine. - 2012. -№7.- C. 101-103.
42. Adapted anastomoses of the jejunum in neonates / D.A. Morozov, I.V. Kirillova, Y.P. Gulyaev [et al.] // Children's Surgery. -2009.- №2.-C. 23-28.
43. Surgery of congenital small intestine obstruction / D.A. Morozov, Y.V. Filippov, S.Y. Gorodkov [et al.] // Russian Bulletin of paediatric surgery, anaesthesiology and resuscitation. - 2011. - № 2. -P. 21-29.
44. Entero- and colostomy in the treatment of malformations and diseases of the gastrointestinal tract in newborns and early infants / V.A. Novozhilov, Y.A. Kozlov, A.A. Kashitsyna [et al.] // Siberian Medical Journal. - 2010. - № 3. - P. 112-114.
45. Long-term results of treatment of children with congenital obstruction of the digestive tract / V.V. Novosad, V.I. Kovalchuk, I.V. Kumova, A.K. Grib // News of Surgery. Novosad, V.I. Kovalchuk, I.V. Kumova, A.K. Grib // News of Surgery. - 2009. - T. 17. - №2.-C. 71-76.
46. Intensive care of newborns with malformations of the gastrointestinal tract and high risk of purulent-septic complications / A.M. Obedin, A.E. Alexandrov, I.V. Kirgizov [et al] //Children's Surgery.-2013.- № 1.-S. 19-21.
47. Olkhova, E.B.. Syndrome of hyperechogenic intestinal contents in newborns / E.B. Olkhova // Radiology-practice. - 2010. - № 5. -C. 417.
48. Parishkov, V.V.. Surgical tactics in acute abdominal pathology in newborns / V.V. Parishkov, A.C. Zheleznov, N.V. Kozulina [et al. Parishkov, A.C. Zhelezhnov, N.V. Kozulina [et al] // Russian Bulletin of paediatric surgery, anaesthesiology and resuscitation. - 2010. - № 1 - C. 54-57.
49. Short bowel syndrome in newborns / D.R. Pogosova, N.M. Rostovtsev, P.G. Baboshko, V.N. Bazaliy // Paediatric Bulletin of the Southern Urals. - 2018. - № 2. - C. 86-92.
50. Clinical efficacy of lagtarocentesis and peritoneal drainage in the treatment of GI perforations in newborns / V.V. Podkamenev. Podkamenev, V.A. Novozhilov, D.V. Timofeev, A.B. Podkamenev // Bulletin of the East-Siberian Scientific Centre SB RAMS. - 2005. -№ 7.-C. 96-100.
51. Popov, F.B. Treatment of newborns and children of the first months of life with small intestinal stoma: author's disc. .... Cand. of medical sciences : 14.00.35 / Popov Fedor Borisovich. - St. Petersburg, 2004. - 17 c.
52. PortnowA. Congenital intestinal obstruction. // Diseases of the gastrointestinal tract (gastroenterology). Last revision:21.11.2021.
53. Prutkin, M.E. Parenteral nutrition of newborns. Methodological materials / M.E.

Prutkin, A.I. Chubarova, D.S. Kryuchko; ed. by H.H. Volodin. Volodin. - M., 2014. - 52 c.
54. Treatment of intestinal atresia in children / G.N.Rumyantseva, Y.F. Brevdo, Y.G. Portenko [et al] // Bulletin of Russian State Medical University. - 2010. - № 3. - C. 41.
55. The structure of causes of lethal outcomes in newborns with surgical pathology / V. A. Savvina, A. R. Varfolomeev, V. N. Nikolaev //Perinatology and neonatology on the materials of dissertations. - Practical Medicine, 2013. -T .06. -#13 . - URL: http ://pmarchive.ru/struktura-prichin-letalnyx-isxodov-u-novorozhdennyx-s-xirurgicheskoj-patologiej/ (date of address: 25. 11. 2013)
56. Congenital intestinal obstruction. Choice of surgical tactics and intestinal suture technique / V.A. Savvina, A.R. Varfolomeev, M.E. Okhlopkov, V.N. Nikolaev // Far Eastern Medical Journal. -2012.-№4.-C. 3740.
57/Pozdozhnya enteroplasty, as cnoci6 of primary treatment, in newborns with proximal atresia of the ileum / O.K. Slepov, M.Y. Migur, O.P. Ponomarenko [et al.] //Ch1rurPya dityachohovhku. - 2018.- T. 4. - № 61. - C. 87-92. - URL: https://doi.org/10.15574/PS.2018.61.87
58 . Slepov O.K., Migur M.Y., Soroka V.P. Xipypri chenelzhuvannya low! at birth obstruction of the small intestine in newborns / O.K. Slepov, M.Y. Migur, V.P. Soroka. P. Soroka // Xipypria dityachogo v.ku. - 2017. - T. 2. - № 55. - C. 70-75. - URL: httpshttps://doi.org/10.15574/PS.2017.55.70doi.org/10.15574/PS.2017.55.70
59 Slepov O. K., Migur M. Y., Zhuravel A. O. Risk factors and !xvpliv on the results of X1 Surgical treatment of low! at birth obstruction of the small intestine in newborn children / O. K., Migur M. Yu. K. Slepov, M. Y. Migur, A. O. Zhuravel // Perinatology and Paediatrics. - 2017. -T. 2. - № 70. - C. 108-112. - URL: httpshttps://doi.org/10.15574/PP.2017.70.108doi.org/10.15574/PP.2017.70.108
60 . Smirnova, A.Yu. Prenatal diagnosis of congenital malformations of the foetus and intrauterine correction of their complications: autoref. diss. . Cand. med. sciences: 14.00.01 / Smirnova Angelika Yuryevna. - Vladivostok, 2009. - 25 c.
61 Solodchuk, O.N. Factors in the formation of dynamic clinical obstruction in premature infants / O.N. Solodchuk, E.P. Sitnikova, A.N. Morugina // Modern Technologies in Medicine. -2009.-№2.-C. 7678.
62 . Dynamic intestinal obstruction in premature infants / O.N. Solodchuk, E.P. Sitnikova, S.A. Petrova [et al] // Voprosy pediatric nutrition. - 2009. - T. 7. - № 2. - C. 76-78.
63 .Sukhotnik, I.G. Short bowel syndrome in children / I.G. Sukhotnik // Russian Herald of paediatric surgery, anaesthesiology and resuscitation. -2017. - T. 7. - № 3. - C. 99-116.
64 Titchenko, L. I. The importance of prenatal ultrasound screening in the detection of congenital malformations / L. I. Titchenko // Russian Herald of Obstetrician and Gynaecologist. - 2006. - T. 6. - № 1. - C. 25-29.
65 . Filippov, Yu. V. Primary adapted intestinal anastomosis in jejunal atresia with

apple peel syndrome / Yu. V. Filippov, D. A. Morozov // Children's Surgery. - 2007. - № 5. - C. 50-51.
66 . Fofanov A.D. Some aspects of surgical treatment of congenital intestinal obstruction in children / A.D. Fofanov // Surgery of Childhood. - 2012. - № 1. - C.49-58.
67 Fofanov, A. D. Intestinal stomas as a stage of surgical treatment of congenital and acquired abdominal pathology in children / A. D. Fofanov, V. A. Fofanov, R. I. Nikiforuk // Surgery of Childhood. - 2014. - № 1-2. - C. 32-37.
68 . Significance of rationally applied high eunostomies in nursing children after small intestine resection / M. G. Chepurnoy, G. I. Chepurnoy, V. B. Katsupeev [et al.] // Medical Bulletin of the North Caucasus.- 2014. - T. 9. - № 1.- C. 13-15.
69 . Shamsiev A.M., Oripov F.S.Epidemiological and morphological characteristics of congenital small intestinal obstruction in newborns / A. M. Shamsiev, F. S. Oripov //Biology va tibbiyot muammolari. - 2018. - №2 (100)- C. 131-133.
70 .Results of surgical treatment of children with small intestine atresia leading to the development of short bowel syndrome / T. N. Shishkina, I. V. Kirgizov, I. A. Shishkin, A. B. Shakhtarin // Children's Surgery. - 2014. - № 1. - C. 19-21.
71 . Shishko, G. A. Parenteral nutrition in newborns / G. A. Shishko, Y. A. Ustinovich. - M.: 2013. - C. 1-12.
72 Ergashev, N.S. Diagnosis and treatment of congenital intestinal obstruction in newborns / N.S. Ergashev, J.B. Sattarov // Modern Medicine: Current Issues. - 2013. - № 25. - C. 58-65.
73 . Antenatal diagnosis of surgical pathology of the fetus according to the data of the National Centre of Medicine of Yakutsk. Yakutsk / V.A. Savvina, M.E. Okhlopkova, JI.B. Gotovtseva [et al] // Far Eastern Medical Journal. - 2003. - № 4. - C. 72-75.
74 .Abdelmohsen S.M, Osman M.A. (2017). Multiple Ileal Atresia with total Colonic Atresia, A Case Report. Madridge J. Case Rep Stud. 1(1): 1619. https://doi.org/10.18689/mjcrs-1000104
75 .Aboalazayem A,Ragab M,Magdy A,Bahaaeldin K,Shalaby A.Outcome of Tapering Enteroplasty in Managing Jejunoileal Atresia.J. Indian Assoc Pediatr. Surg. 2022 Nov-Dec;27(6):666-669. doi: 10.4103/jiaps.jiaps_1_22. Epub 2022 Nov 14.PMid: 36714492
76 .Ademuyiwa A.O., Sowande O.A., Ijaduola T.K., O. Adejuyigbe Determinants of mortality in neonatal intestinal obstruction in He Ife, NigeriaAfr. J. Pediatr. Surg. 2009. Vol. 6, № 1.P.11-13.
77 .Ademuyiwa O.A. Determinants of mortality in neonatal intestinal obstruction in He Ife, Nigeria. Afr. J. Paediatr. Surg. 2009. Vol. 6. P. 11-13.
78 .Aggerwal N, Sugandhi N, Kour H, Chakraborty G, Acharya SK, Jadhav A, Bagga D. (2019). Total intestinal atresia: Revisiting the pathogenesis of congenital atresias. J. Indian Assoc Pediatr Surg. 24: 303
306. https://doi.org/10.4103/jiaps.JIAPS 204 18 ;PMid: 31571767 PMCid:PMC6752068.

79. Aguayo P., Ostlie D. Duodenal and intestinal atresia and stenosis.In Holcomb G., Murphy P., Ostlie D.: Aschcrafts Pediatric Surgery, 6th ed. Elsevier Saunders; 2014.
80. AhmaduB.U. etal. Neonatal intestinal obstruction secondary to mid-gut volvulus complicated by bowel gangrene in a neonate with ileal atresia. Clin. Med. Res. 2013. Vol. 2. P. 101-104.
81. Almoutaz A. Different surgical techniques in management of small intestinal atresia in high risk neonates. Ann. Pediatr. Surg. 2009. Vol. 5, № 1.P. 31-35.
82. Ameh E.A., Ayeni M.A., Kache S.A., Mshelbwala P.M. Role of damage control enterostomy in management of children with peritonitis from acute intestinal disease. J. Pediatr. Surg. 2013. Vol. 10, № 4. P. 315-319.
83. Anatol T.I., Hariharan S. Congenital intestinal obstruction in a Caribbean country. Int Surg. 2009. Vol. 94, № 3. P. 212-216.
84. Aranda A. Neonatal Intestinal Anastomosis Using a 5 mm Laparoscopic Stapler. *J. Laparoendosc Adv Surg Tech A*. 2019;29:579-581.
85. AzizD.A., SehatS.I., OsmanM., Zaki F.M. Neonatal intestinal obstruction secondary to a floppy Meckel's diverticulum successfully treated by minimal access surgery. BMJ Case Reports. 2012. http://www.researchgate.net.
86. Babaei H., Ahmadipour S.H., Mohamadimoghadam J. The study of newborns with congenital gastrointestinal tract obstruction. J. Krishna Institute Med. Sciences University. 2014. Vol. 3, № 2. P. 101-106.
87. Balanescu R., Topor L., Stoica I., Moga A., Associated type III B and type IV multiple intestinal atresia in a paediatric patient. Chirurgia. 2013. Vol. 3.P. 407410.
88. Barakat N.A., Maati S.H., Nutritional and surgical management of short bowel syndrome in neonates. Res. J. Med. Med. Sci. 2009. Vol. 4.P. 220-223.
89. Bayol N.U. et al. Documentation of small intestinal atresias: a single institution experience in Turkey (22 cases). Turk. J. Med. Sci. 2011. Vol.41, No.6. P. 10651069.
90. BestK.E., TennantP.W., Addor M.C. et al.Epidemiology of small intestinal atresia in Europe: a register-based study. Arch. Dis. Child. Fetal Neonatal Ed. 2012. Vol. 97, № 5. P. F353-358.
91. BlaszczynskiM., PorzucekW., BecelaP., Gadzinowski J. T-tube enterostomy in surgical management of emergency cases in neonate. Arch. Perin. Med.2011.Vol. 13, № 2. P. 93-96.
92. Boo Y., Goedeke J., Engel V., Muenstere O. A case report of laparoscopic
93. Bracho-BlanchetE., Gonzalez-ChavezA., Davila-Perez R. et al. Prognostic factors related to mortality in newborns with jejuno-ileal atresia. Cir. Cir. 2012. Vol. 80, № 4. P. 345-351.
94. Burjonrappa S.C. Crete E., Bouchard S. Prognostic factors in jejuno-ileal atresia. Pediatr. Surg. Int. 2009. Vol. 25. P. 795-798.
95. Burjonrappa S.C., Crete E., Bouchard S. Comparative outcomes in intestinal atresia: a clinical outcome and pathophysiology analysis. Pediatr. Surg. Int. 2011. Vol. 27, № 4. P. 437-442.
96. BurkiT., KihoL., Scheimberg I. et al. Neonatal functional intestinal obstruction

and the presence of severely immature ganglion cells on rectal biopsy: a 6yearexperience. Pediatr. Surg. Int. 2011. Vol. 27, № 5. P. 487-490.
97. Charles W.H., Stanley T.L., Sani Z.Y. et al. Enteroplasty for Complicated Meconium Ileus. Curr. Pediatr. Rev. 2010. Vol. 6, № 4. - P. 234-236.
98. Charlorin P, Louima O, Pierre GS, Peigne R, Bowder A, Grazia Maria A, Sylvio A. (2020). Use of feeding jejunostomy in a type IV jejuno-ileal atresia in a low-income country. Journal of Pediatric Surgery Case Reports. https://doi.org/10.1016Zi.epsc.2020.101580
99. Chirdan L.B., Uba A.F., Pam S.D. (2004). Intestinal atresia: management problems in a developing country. Pediatr Surg Int. 20:834837. https://doi.org/10.1007/s00383-004-1152-4. PMid:15138787
100. Dao D.T., Demehri F.R., Barnewolt C.E. et al. A new variant of type III jejunoileal atresia. J PediatrSurg. 2019;54(6): 1257-1260. https://doi.org/10.1016/j. jpedsurg.2019.02.003.
101. Das P.C., Shrecdhara K.A. Apple peel jejunal atresia in a neonate: a rare cause of intestinal obstruction. Int. J. Biomed. Res. 2012. №3.P. 114-115.
102. Dewberry L.C., Hilton S.A., Vuille-Dit-Bille R.N., Liechty K.W.. Is tapering enteroplasty an alternative to resection of dilated bowel in small intestinal atresia? J. Surg Res. 2020. 246:1-5. doi: 10.1016/j.jss.2019.08.014
103. Diagnosis of Fetal Abnormalities. G. Pilu, K. Nicolaides, R. Ximenes, P. Jianty. - London: ISOUG and Fetal Medicine Foundation, 2002. - 135 p.
104. Duodenal atresia repair in a neonate using a novel miniature stapling device. Int J. of Surg Case Reports. 2017;30:31-33.
105. Efrati O. et al. Meconium ileus in patients with cystic fibrosis is not a risk factor for clinical deterioration and survival: the Israeli Multicenter Study. J.Pediatr. Gastroenterol. Nutr. 2010. Vol. 50, № 2. P. 173-178.
106. Ekenze S.O., Ibeziako S.N., Ezomike U.O.. Trends in neonatal intestinal obstruction in a developing country, 1996-2005. World J. Surg. 2007.Vol. 31, № 12. P. 2405-2409.
107. Eltayeb A.A. Different surgical techniques in management of small intestinal atresia in high risk neonates.J. Pediatr. Pediatr. Surg. 2009. - № 5.P. 31-35.
108. Fragoso A., Ortiz R., Hernandez F., Olivares P., Martinez L., Tovar J.A. Defective upper gastrointestinal function after repair of combined esophageal and duodenal atresia. J. Pediatr. Surg. 2015; 50 (4): 531-4.
109. Gfroerer S., Fiegel H., Ramachandran P. et al. Changes of smooth muscle contractile filaments in small bowel atresia. World J. Gastroenterol. - 2012. Vol. 18, №24. P. 3099-3104.
110. Ghafouri-Taleghani F. T., N. Abdolreza., Ahmadreza Z. Long term clinical outcome of small intestinal atresia in children, a single centre experience. Govaresh. 2015. Vol. 31, № 12. P. 2405-2409.
111. BertholdK., OlivierG., JoanneH. et al. Guidelines on Pediatric Parenteral Nutrition of the European Society of Pediatric Gastroenterology, Hepatology and

Nutrition (ESPGHAN) and the European Society for Clinical Nutrition and Metabolism (ESPEN), Supported by the European Society of Pediatric Research (ESPR). J. Pediatr. Gastroenterol. Nutr. - 2005. - No. 41, Suppl. 2. - P. 81 - 87.

112. H., Lane G.J., Miyano T. Laparoscopy-assisted surgery for prenatally diagnosed small bowel atresia: simple, safe, and virtually scar free. J. Pediatr Surg. 2004;39:1815-1818.

113. Henderson L.B., Doshi V.K., Blackman S.M. et al. Variation in MSRA modifies risk of neonatal intestinal obstruction in cystic fibrosis. PLoS Genet. 2012. Vol. 8, № 3. http://www.biomedsearch.com.

114. Hill S., Koontz C.S., Langness S.M., Wulkan M.L.. Laparoscopic versus open repair of congenital duodenal obstruction in infants. J. Laparoendosc. Adv. Surg. Tech. A. 2011; 21 (10): 961-3.

115. Hyseni N. et al. Successful treatment of multiple jejuno-ileal atresia by four primary anastomosis and trans anastomotic silastic stents. J.K.Sci. - 2009.Vol. 11.P.136-138.

116. Imran M.U., Rehman T. Wahed Sigmoid Atresia. A rare cause of neonatal intestinal obstruction. J.KUST Med. 2009. Vol.1, No.2. P. 71-72.

117. Islam S.S., Faisal I., Ahmed M. Etiology and treatment outcome of neonatal intestinal obstruction in a tertiary hospital. J. Ped. Sur. Bang. 2010.Vol. 1,№1.P.30-36.

118. JawadM, KlafkowskiG, LenneyW, Gilchrist F.J.Intestinal obstruction secondary to adhesions in an infant with cystic fibrosis. BMJCaseReports. 2013. http://casereports.bmj.com/content/2013/bcr-2013-0104444.

119. Jeanty C., Frayer E.A., Page R., Langenburg S.Neonatal ovarian torsion complicated by intestinal obstruction and perforation, and review of the literature. J. Pediatr. Surg. 2010. Vol. 45, № 6. - P. 5-9.

120. John G., S.O. Choi., Raffensperger M.D. Childrens surgery: a worldwide history. PediatricSurgeryBooks .McFarland.2013. http://www.pediatricsurgerybooks.com.

121. Jung E. Primary segmental volvulus of the ileum mimicking meconium plug syndrome. J. Korean Surg. Soc. - 2011.-Vol. 80. - P . 85-87.

122. Khalaf A.A., Al-Obaidy M.A. Jejunoileal Atresia A study of 60 cases in children welfare teaching hospital. J. Fac. Med. Baghda. 2010. Vol. 52, № 3. P. 248-245.

123. Kozlov Y., Novogilov V., Podkamenev A., Weber I. Stapled bowel anastomoses in newborn surgery. Eur. J. Pediatr. Surg. 2013. Vol. 23, № 1.P. 6366.

124. Li B, Chen W, Wang S, et al. Laparoscopy-assisted surgery for neonatal intestinal atresia and stenosis: a report of 35 cases. J.Pediatr. Surg. Int. 2012; 28(12):1225-1228.

125. Machmouchi M. New successful one-step surgical repair for apple peel atresia. Open Access Surg. - 2011. Vol. 4. P. 53-56.

126. Millar A.J.W. Short Bowel Syndrome.2011. http://global-help.org.

127. Mirza B., N. Bux II. Multiple Congenital Segmental Dilatations of Colon.

Neonatal Surg. 2012. Vol. 1, №3. P.5-8.
128. Mitul AR. "Congenital Neonatal Intestinal Obstruction". J. ofNenatal Surgery. 2016. Oct-Dec; 5(4): 41.
129. Mohamed S.Sh., Kamal K, Mohamed S.Sh., Gregor W. Intestinal malrotation and volvulus in infants and children. BMJ. 2013. Vol. 347.
130. Mohammad I., Rehman H.U., Rehman I.U.. Outcome of Bishop Koop Procedure in neonatal Jejenoileal atresias: A Retrospective Analysis. Korean Med. Journal. 2011. № 3. P. 52-56.
131. Morris G., Kennedy A. Jr., Cochran W. Small bowel congenital anomalies. A review and update. CurrGastroenterol Rep. 18(4): 16, 2016. doi: 10.1007/s11894-016-0490-4
132. Nusinovich Y, Revenis M, Torres C. Long-term outcomes for infants with intestinal atresia studied at Children's National Medical Centre. J. Ped. Gastroenterol. Nutrit. 2013. Vol. 57, № 3. P. 324-329.
133. Osifo O.D. Neonatal intestinal obstruction in Benin, Nigeria. Afr. J. Paediatr. Surg. 2009. Vol. 6, № 2. P. 98-101.
134. Osifo O.D. Management of intestinal atresia: Challenges and outcomes in a resource-scarce region. J. Surg. Pract. 2009. Vol. 13.P. 36-41.
135. Osifo O.D., M.E. Ovueni. The Prevalence, patterns, and causes of deaths of surgical neonates at two African referral pediatric surgical centres. Ann. Pediatr. Surg. 2009. - Vol. 5, № 3. P. 194-199.
136. Ozturk H., Gedik S. et al. A comprehensive analysis of 51 neonates with congenital intestinal atresia. Saudi Med. J. - 2007. Vol. 28. - P. 1050-1054.
137. Paradiso V.F., Briganti V., Oriolo L. et al. Meconium obstruction in absence of cystic fibrosis in low birth weight infants: an emerging challenge from increasing survival. Ital. J. Pediatr. 2011. Vol. 37. P. 55.
138. Patel R.V., Shepherd G., Kumar H., N. Patwardhan. Neonatal Currarino's syndrome presenting as intestinal obstruction. BMJCase Reports.2013. http://www.researchgate.net.
139. Patil V.K Neonatal adrenal hemorrhage presenting as intestinal obstruction. Ind. Pediatr. 2011. Vol. 48, № 9. P. 738-739.
140. Polin R., Spitzer A. Fetal and neonatal secrets. St. Louis: Mosby, 2007. P. 428.
141. Puralingegowda A.K., Mohanty P.K., Razak A. et al. Neonatal intestinal obstruction secondary to a small bowel duplication cyst. BMJ Case Reports. 2014. http://casereports.bmj.com.
142. Raghu S. Sadashiva R., Kishan B.S. Primary segmental volvulus mimicking ileal atresia. J. Neonat. Surg. 2013. № 2. P. 6-9.
143. Rathod K.J., Mohd Z., Kanojia R., Rao K.L.. Segmental ileal dilatation: an unsuspected cause of neonatal intestinal obstruction. Trop. Gastroenterol. 2012. Vol. 33, №2. P.143-146.
144. Rode H., Numanoglu A. Diagnosis and management. J. Pediatr. Surg. 2009. Vol. 8. P. 405-414.

145. Rothenberg S.S. Laparoscopic duodenoduodenostomy for duodenal obstruction in infants and children. J. Pediatr. Surg. 2002; 37: 1088-9.
146. Saha H, Halder A, Chatterjee U, et al. Clinicopathological study of intestinal smooth muscles, interstitial cells of Cajal and enteric neurons in neonatal jejunoileal atresia with special reference to muscle morphometry. J. Pediatr.Surg. 2019;54(11):2291-2299. https://doi.org/10.1016Zj. jpedsurg.2019.06.003
147. Saha S., Koner H., Saha K. et al. A neonatal intestinal obstruction with unusual presentation. J. Ind. Med. Assoc. 2006. - Vol. 104, № 5. P. 267-268.
148. Santulli T.V., Blanc W.A. Congenital atresia of intestine: Pathogenesis and treatment. Ann. Surg. 1961. Vol. 154. P. 939.
149. Sato K., Uchida H., Tanaka Y. et al. Stapled intestinal anastomosis is a simple and reliable method for management of intestinal caliber discrepancy in children. J. Pediatr. Surg. Int. 2012. Vol. 28. P. 893-898.
150. Shakya V.C., Agrawal Ch.S. Management of jejunoilealatresias: an experience in eastern Nepal. BMC Surg. 2010. Vol. 10. P. 35-39.
151. Sinha Sh., Sarin Y.K.. Outcome of jejuno-ileal atresia associated with intraoperative finding of volvulus of small bowel. J. Neonat. Surg. 2012. Vol. 1, № 3. P. 38.
152. Springer Sh.C. Bowel obstruction in the Newborn. Medscape Reference. 2011. http://y/emedicine.medscape.com.
153. Stollman T.N., BlaauwI.D., WijnenM.H.et al. Decreased mortality but increased morbidity in neonates with jejunoileal atresia; a study of 114 cases over a 34-year period. J. Pediatr. Surg. 2009. Vol. 44. P. 217-221.
154. Tsai L.Y., Hsieh W.S., Chen C.Y. et al. Distinct clinical characteristics of patients with congenital duodenal obstruction in a medical centre in Taiwan. J. Pediatr. Neonatology. 2010. Vol. 51, № 6. P. 343-346.
155. VinocurD.N.,Lee R.L.. Eisenberg Neonatal intestinal obstruction. AJR. 2012. Vol. 198, № 1. P. Wl-10.
156. Walk C., Meagher D., Christian J., Barnett S., Pence J., Chaudhary M.,William J., Cochran M.D. Geisinger ClinicOverview of Congenital Gastrointestinal Anomalies. Jejunoileal atresia. Neonat. Surg. 2012. Vol. 1, № 3. P. 38.
157. Yamataka A., Koga H., Shimotakahara A. et al. Laparoscopy-assisted surgery for prenatally diagnosed small bowel atresia: Simple, safe, and virtually scar free. J. Pediatr Surg. 2004;39(12):1815-1818.https://doi.org/10.1016/j. jpedsurg.2004.08.029.
158. Yang S., Wang M., Shen C. Bowel plication in neonatal high jejunal atresia. Medicine. 2019;98(19):e15459. https://doi.org/10.1097/ MD.0000000000015459.
159. Martinez-Ferro M., Rothenberg S., St Peter S., Bignon H., Holcomb G. Laparoscopic treatment of post necrotising enterocolitis colonic strictures. J. Laparoendosc Adv. Surg. Tech. A.2010;20:477-480.

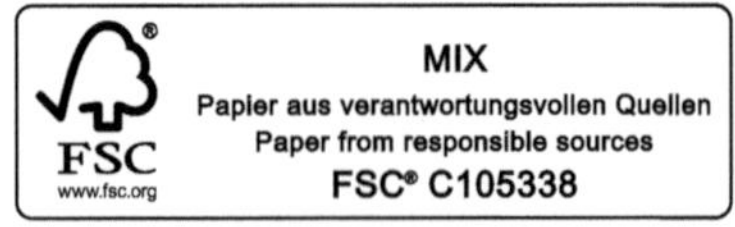

Printed by Books on Demand GmbH, Norderstedt / Germany